CABIN FEVER

SocietyNow

SocietyNow: short, informed books, explaining why our world is the way it is, now.

The *SocietyNow* series provides readers with a definitive snapshot of the events, phenomena and issues that are defining our twenty-first century world. Written leading experts in their fields and publishing as each subject is being contemplated across the globe, titles in the series offer a thoughtful, concise and rapid response to the major political and economic events and social and cultural trends of our time.

SocietyNow makes the best of academic expertise accessible to a wider audience, to help readers untangle the complexities of each topic and make sense of our world the way it is, now.

CABIN FEVER

Surviving Lockdown in the Coronavirus Pandemic

BY

PAUL CRAWFORD
University of Nottingham, UK

JAMIE ORION CRAWFORD
Montreal, Canada

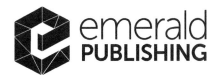

United Kingdom – North America – Japan – India
Malaysia – China

Emerald Publishing Limited
Howard House, Wagon Lane, Bingley BD16 1WA, UK

First edition 2021

Reprints and permissions service
Contact: permissions@emeraldinsight.com

British Library Cataloguing in Publication Data
A catalogue record for this book is available from the British Library

ISBN: 978-1-80071-355-0 (Print)
ISBN: 978-1-80071-352-9 (Online)
ISBN: 978-1-80071-354-3 (Epub)

ISOQAR certified
Management System,
awarded to Emerald
for adherence to
Environmental
standard
ISO 14001:2004.

Certificate Number 1985
ISO 14001

INVESTOR IN PEOPLE

To all who experienced the greatest confinement in history

CONTENTS

ABOUT THE AUTHORS

Paul Crawford is the world's first Professor of Health Humanities, pioneering the field and launching multiple new research, educational and practice initiatives worldwide. He directs the Centre for Social Futures at the Institute of Mental Health at the University of Nottingham, UK. Co-directs the Health Humanities Research Priority Area at the University of Nottingham. He is also an Adjunct Professor at the University of Canberra. His recent publications include *Health Humanities* (Palgrave, 2015), *Humiliation* (Emerald, 2019), *The Routledge Companion to Health Humanities* (Routledge, 2020) and *Florence Nightingale at Home* (Palgrave, 2020). He is also the editor of the Emerald *Arts for Health* Series (Emerald) for the general reader and Joint Editor-in-Chief for *The Palgrave Encyclopedia of Health Humanities* (Springer, in press).

Jamie Orion Crawford is a data analyst and researcher based in Montreal, Canada. He is experienced in analysing diverse data from a wide range of industrial contexts – most recently the music industry for Wavo.me. He has contributed editorial advice to various publications including Crawford et al. (eds) *The Routledge Companion to Health Humanities* (Routledge, 2020) and Crawford et al. *Florence Nightingale at Home* (Palgrave, 2020). This is his first co-authored book project.

ACKNOWLEDGEMENTS

We wish to thank the University of Nottingham, the Wellcome Collection and the British Library in providing excellent online archives and resources.

PC: Special thanks to my wife, Fei-Chi, whose absence during lockdown made my heart grow fonder still; to Jamie for agreeing to counter my isolation by co-authoring this book; to Ruby and Owen for the occasional visits to my urban desert island and virtual hugs during shielding; to my brother Mark and his wife Christina who kept me sane by phone; to friends, neighbours and colleagues for their generous relief missions, bringing food, newspapers and 3D humanity. The 2 metre divide always seemed so much more.

JOC: Special thanks to my love, Andrea, for putting up with me (in general, but especially during lockdown) and to Brian and Mairi for allowing us to isolate ourselves at Komo cottage; to my dad for his lively debate and for this wonderful opportunity to write a book together; to the strongest person I know, my mum, who kept my spirits high with virtual visits to my island in Animal Crossing; to my grandparents, Orion and Eunice, whose regular video updates never failed to make me smile; and finally, to Josh, Will, Justin and Pierre for providing much needed comic relief.

1

THE GREATEST CONFINEMENT
IN HISTORY

This short book discusses the origins, definitions, social and cross-cultural history of the popularly framed condition of cabin fever in relation to what became the greatest confinement in history resulting from the coronavirus pandemic in 2020 (henceforth simply referred to as 'the pandemic') as governments imposed lockdown measures – e.g. quarantines, stay-at-home orders, shelter-in-place orders, shutdowns and curfews – to slow the spread of the virus. Indeed, it is estimated that around 4.2 billion, 54% of the global population, were subject to complete or partial lockdowns at the height of the pandemic (IEA, 2020). The book also examines creative individual and community responses to mass enforced isolation in its various forms. In the former, engagement and relationships may be limited, or at best, achieved only in virtual contexts such as through social media. For groups or communities, direct, physical connection presents a different challenge, not least achieving distance from others or wanting a break from them.

The notion of cabin fever and related terms, such as going stir-crazy (derived from the use of *stir* to mean 'prison'), has emerged in media representation and raises the very real question of how strongly this features in the current pandemic (Henley, 2020; Kanthor, 2020; Sims, 2020). In an anecdotal report on early lockdown measures, British tourist Peter Grantham commented:

> *We were also worried about people's mental health. People had been there for a month. And it was a bit of like, kind of, cabin fever I could see happening to a few individuals on site.*
>
> (Grantham, 2020)

Are people losing their minds during the great confinement? Are they suffering from cabin fever, going stir-crazy and, if so, how is that evident? How are people managing in the confines of their homes, however large or small, whether in apartments or houses with gardens for weeks, if not months, at a time? Which is worse, to be left on your own at this time or subject to close quarters with other cohabitees, whether members of family, friends or even strangers? These and many other questions need considering if we are to begin to determine how far the concept of cabin fever applies in this case.

During the writing of this book the first author remained in lockdown in a detached urban house with access to a garden in the United Kingdom, with his two younger children staying with their mother and his wife stranded in Taiwan. His son, the second author, took to a remote cottage along the Ottawa River in Canada with his partner who captured their isolation in a painting. In the image, the cloned, replicated images of themselves appear to form a community against a wintry desolation (Fig. 1.1).

Families around the world found themselves within a single dwelling or living separately in different accommodation. The lived circumstances for individuals, families and non-family groups in this period has been diverse, but all those subject

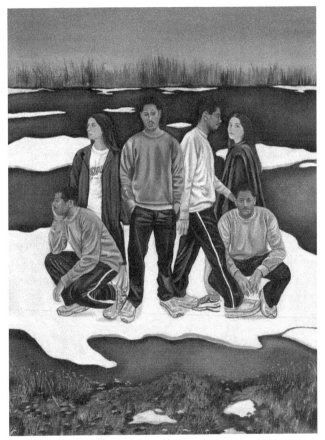

Fig. 1.1. 'On Ice' by Andrea Wilkin.

to the great confinement, being told stay at home and follow social distancing rules, would have likely experienced a tension between indoor and outdoor life, making difficult decisions based on their work and the need to shop for food, exercise or support others to leave the perceived safety of their homes. In normal circumstances, except perhaps in war zones or areas of high crime, people would have passed back and forth across the threshold of their dwellings without a second thought. In the

ravages of the pandemic, each domestic threshold became a
borderland of decisions and risk. The outside, social world of
the rampaging virus became a palpable and very real threat.
Many would have experienced the kind of hesitancy between
entrapment and escape conjured up in Holly St. John Bergon's
poem *Cabin Fever* (2009). In her poem, she captures the tension between a call to leave and desire to stay, between the
threat of both interior and exterior spaces (Fig. 1.2).

> *In cabin fever dreams, I've lost my way.*
>
> *The wind sighs, Leave, and opens wide the door.*
>
> *Although I want to go, I think I'll stay.*

Never before in human history have so many people been
confined to their homes as they have been with the outbreak
and spread of the pandemic in 2020, all experiencing the
uncomfortable threshold palpable between the inside and

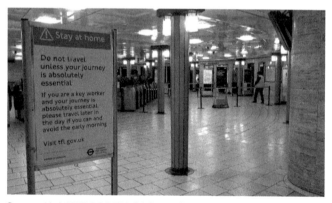

Source: Kwh1050 / CC BY-SA (https://creativecommons.org/licenses/
by-sa/4.0); https://upload.wikimedia.org/wikipedia/commons/3/35/
Piccadilly_Circus_station_during_London_COVID-19_lockdown._
Sign.jpg.

**Fig. 1.2. Stay at Home: Piccadilly Circus Station during
London COVID-19 Lockdown.**

outside in Bergon's poem. In this bicentenary year of one of the greatest contributors to public health, Florence Nightingale, billions of people faced an unprecedented scourge that left them self-isolating in their homes through either personal choice or the mandates of state governments globally (Sandford, 2020).

Preventing contagion at home and in hospitals, alongside championing public sanitation and the use of statistics to track disease and mortality, had been at the heart of Nightingale's work. She also suffered prolonged periods of seclusion at home for much of the rest of her life after contracting brucellosis from infected milk while attending to wounded soldiers from the Crimean War (1854–1856). That said, the greatest part of Nightingale's scholarly and epistolary efforts to improve public health were achieved while housebound, as an invalid working from her bed (Crawford, Greenwood, Bates, & Memel, 2020b). Her productivity over many years was remarkable despite the confinement that many in lockdown have experienced. She did not find being a prisoner at home at all easy despite the luxury of receiving financial support from her wealthy father. In a draft letter to the crown princess of Prussia in 1861, she writes:

> *I have passed the last four years between four walls,*
> *only varied to other four walls once a year; and*
> *I believe there is no prospect but of my health*
> *becoming ever worse and worse till the hour of my*
> *release.*

(McDonald, 2011, p. 621)

Two hundred years after Nightingale's birth in 1820, governments around the world are revisiting her substantial public health efforts, not least in advocating hand-washing and ventilating accommodation to reduce contagion, in their own response to the current pandemic. Voluntary and involuntary sequestering in people's homes, alone or with family members, friends or even strangers, to halt the spread of the virus and the impact on limited health services has provoked anticipation across all major organisations and bodies, not least the World Health Organization (WHO, 2020), as to the mental health challenges of this radical social change. As Holmes et al. (2020) note, social isolation and loneliness are 'strongly associated with anxiety, depression, self-harm, and suicide attempts across the life-span'. Furthermore, the authors point out that isolation is exacerbated by the 'entrapment' brought by the social distancing initiatives to deal with the pandemic. For those confined to apartments this seclusion was particularly challenging. Some relief could be found on balconies as in the following image from Belgrade, Serbia (Fig. 1.3).

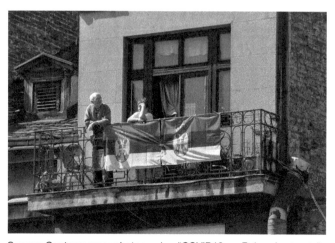

Source: Contemporary photography: "COVID19 on Belgrade streets" by SaraRistic is licensed under CC BY-NC-SA 2.0. https://search.creativecommons.org/photos/a7f5466a-01dc-4715-a7cc-dbafcd90aa9b.

Fig. 1.3. Lockdown.

SOCIAL ISOLATION

Social isolation can be defined as 'a deprivation of social connectedness' or 'the inadequate quality and quantity of social relations with other people at the different levels where human interaction takes place (individual, group, community and the larger social environment)' (Zavaleta, Samuel, & Mills, 2014, p. 5). Such isolation can be considered to provoke or lead to the distressing emotional state of loneliness (see Hawkley & Cacioppo, 2009). There have been a number of scholars down the years who have examined multiple aspects of social isolation and loneliness. David Riesman in his book *The Lonely Crowd* (1950) marked a weakening of autonomy in American society as people became more other-directed or obsessed, with popular culture replicating the 'crowd' and offering a way to escape the 'terror of loneliness' (p. 170). In a further critique of the individualism and isolationism of American society in his book *The Pursuit of Loneliness* (1970), Philip Slater flagged up the dangers succinctly in a short 'cabin fever' story as a preface which starts:

> *Once upon a time there was a man who sought escape from the prattle of his neighbors and went to live alone in a hut he had found in the forest. At first he was content, but a bitter winter led him to cut down the trees around his hut for firewood. The next summer he was hot and uncomfortable because his hut had no shade, and he complained of the harshness of the elements.*

(p. 21)

His isolation brings increasing losses, not least in social perspective. He ends up shooting at intruders and blows off his own foot while sleeping with his gun. In *Bowling Alone*

(2000), Robert D. Putnam extends this concern for the dangers of individualism over community bonds and, more recently, Sherry Turkle interrogates in *Alone Together* (2011) the risk of technologically mediated social interaction, its illusory companionship, and paradoxical heightened connectivity at the same time as increased solitude and loneliness. In the pandemic, the parameters and, indeed, balance between the individual and community, togetherness and loneliness, and online and offline contact are being revisited. Individual isolation or even the softer realm of solitude is being placed under a durative stress test.

According to Wang et al. (2017) social isolation can be determined and measured in terms of the quantity, structure and quality of an individual's social networks and by appraisal of their relationships from emotional and resource perspectives. We may think of resources in terms of individual or ecological social capital or the assets or supports people have access to in themselves or out there in 'society'. A lack of these can damage mental health, not least in depression and suicide. Whereas access to such assets can support or enhance psychological well-being.

MENTAL HEALTH

The burden of mental distress has been endemic to humans long before the emergence of the pandemic. Mental distress, or illness, accounts for the second biggest threat to our financial and social stability behind cardiovascular disease (Centre for Mental Health, 2010; WHO, 2005; Wittchen et al., 2011). In the United Kingdom, mental health has been advanced as pivotal to health overall with the slogan 'no health without mental health' (Department of Health, 2011). For many years now social isolation and social exclusion in societies worldwide have been a cause for concern. Many people feel they no longer belong to a community (Griffin, 2010). Isolation and loneliness appear to be on the rise (Gierveld, Tilburg, & Dykstra, 2018). As indicated by Holt-Lunstad, Smith, and Layton (2010), social isolation leads to higher premature mortality, not least suicide. Importantly, mental health deteriorates with social isolation (Elovainio et al., 2017) and quarantine (Brooks et al., 2020); it often accompanies mental illness (Beutel et al., 2017) and should be further investigated in the context of the pandemic (Durcan, O'Shea, & Allwood, 2020).

Research on the fallout of social isolation adding to the burden of mental health began in earnest around the world in the early months of the pandemic. For example, there have been studies and reports emerging from the United Kingdom (Allington et al., 2020a; Cowan, 2020; Holmes et al., 2020; Marsh, 2020), United States (Li & Schwartzapfel, 2020; Taub, 2020; Well Being Trust, 2020), China (Allen-Ebrahimian, 2020; Li & Gang, 2020; Liu et al., 2020; Xiang et al., 2020), India (Varshney, Parel, Raizada, & Sarin, 2020), Australia (Department of Health, 2020), Brazil (Serafim, Gonçalves, Rocca, & Neto, 2020; Zhang, Wang, Jahanshahi, Li, & Schmitt, 2020), Russia (Gritsenko et al., 2020; Sorokin et al., 2020), Ghana (Gyasi, 2020) and South Africa (Joska et al., 2020). These reveal increased fear, anxiety, depression, loneliness, violence, suicidal thinking and suicide rates.

The magnitude of the impacts appears substantial. For example, Varshney et al. (2020) during the initial stages of the pandemic in India found that around a third of respondents had endured a significant psychological impact. In the United Kingdom, Allington et al. (2020a) in their survey found that 49% were more anxious or depressed than usual, 38% slept less or less well, 35% had eaten more food or less healthy food than normal, 19% drank more alcohol than normal and 19% argued more with their family or housemates than normal. Of particular concern has been the impact on harmful behaviour of suicide and self-harm. This impact is highlighted in early reports from the United Kingdom and United States (see Holmes et al., 2020; Marsh, 2020; Well Being Trust, 2020). A study at University College London, for example, found that 18% of people surveyed in the United Kingdom alone had considered self-harming or killing themselves during lockdown (Marsh, 2020). Even though this survey was self-selecting and promoted by UK Research and Innovation, such indicative figures are worrying.

Another particularly dark consequence to the enforced isolation of lockdown featured in early research has been increased domestic violence (Li & Schwartzapfel, 2020; Taub, 2020) which chimes strongly with the phenomenon of cabin fever. In Christensen's early article on cabin fever (Christensen, 1984), domestic violence is noted as a possible indicator of the condition. Indeed, forcibly 'isolating a person from family and friends' is a tactic commonly used by batterers to establish control and facilitate abuse (WHO, 2012). For women and men subject to domestic violence the experience of cabin fever will be as much about seeking relational escape as that of spatial release.

However, Gunnell et al. (2020) argue that this is not inevitable given national efforts at mitigation. Also, while cabin fever may be a highly plausible driver for increased rates of depression, anxiety and self-harm, other indirect stressors are known such as general economic uncertainty, increased levels of domestic violence as noted above or abuse of children at home. Allen-Ebrahimian (2020) flags up a domestic violence epidemic in China following its lockdown. This corollary of confinement at home is evidenced globally (Graham-Harrison, Giuffrida, Smith, & Ford, 2020). In a most tragic case, two young children were stabbed to death by their father (Karim, 2020). As yet we do not know how far mitigating actions will fully address the mental health challenges of the lockdown. Many commentators are not as sanguine as Gunnell et al. (2020) on this matter. For example, Gregory (2020) reports on how a large number of people are expected to require help following the pandemic in recovering from anxiety, depression and post-traumatic stress disorder.

The likelihood of a significant mental health fallout from the pandemic is further indicated with data emerging only seven weeks into lockdown in the United Kingdom by the mental health charity Sane who reported a 200% increase in calls to their helpline, many of whom were first-time callers (Vincent, 2020). This, among other similar reports, suggests that the isolation behind closed doors is resulting in what, as a folk term, we call cabin fever. A survey that tracks the mood of around 2,000 Britons weekly indicated a significant rise in boredom and fear and a commensurate fall in happiness during lockdown (YouGov, 2020). A Kings' College study identified three groups reacting to life under lockdown as accepting (48%), suffering (44%) and resisting (9%). Of those suffering, 93% reported anxiety and depression, 64% reduced or disrupted sleep, 34% constant thinking about coronavirus and 64% checking of social media on coronavirus daily or more frequently (Allington et al., 2020b).

Although many people found themselves in lockdown in company with friends, partners or other family members, not least children, others will have experienced this alone or in institutions such as care homes where strict quarantine often ruled out family visits. Thousands of these institutions world-wide locked their doors to visitors as in the following image of the Dreamland Nursing Home in India. While the pandemic lockdown lies outside the penal system and the whole business of punishment, it is worth dwelling on the impact of solitary confinement in this case (Fig. 1.4).

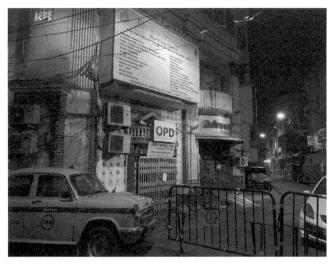

Credit: Indrajit Das / CC BY-SA.

Fig. 1.4. Dreamland Nursing Home.

SOLITARY CONFINEMENT

In 1829, George W. Smith's defence of the system of solitary confinement in the State of Pennsylvania underlined its long-standing, wide use:

> *As a means of mere effectual seclusion from society and the prevention of further injury by prisoners during the period of incarceration, and as a mode of inflicting vindictive punishment, it has been partially practised in almost every nation from the remotest ages.*
>
> (Smith, 1833, p. 7)

However, as society progressed from the nineteenth to the twentieth century, concerns increased about the use of solitary confinement in prisons. In a fairly early text, Nitsche and

Wilmanns (1912) noted both the 'dangers of ennui' and solitary confinement or isolation in prisons, with the latter deemed 'largely responsible for the frequent outbreaks of mental disturbance' (pp. 26–27). In her book, *Solitary Confinement: Social Death and its Afterlives* (2013), 100 years on, Lisa Guenther powerfully presents the continuing damage of social confinement in the US penal system. In particular, she notes the dire impact on a person's psychological, social and 'basic' identity. She writes,

> *There are many ways to destroy a person, but one of the simplest and most devastating is through prolonged solitary confinement. Deprived of meaningful human interaction, otherwise healthy prisoners become unhinged. They see things that do not exist, and they fail to see things that do.*
> (2013, p. xi)

She summarises the universal symptoms of 'anxiety, fatigue, confusion, paranoia, depression, hallucinations, headaches and uncontrollable trembling' (2013, p. xii) (Fig. 1.5).

Guenther goes on to outline how such confinement, often in small spaces, brings a 'social death', and inmates have to learn ways to adjust to the expanse of 'dead time' that lies ahead. The deleterious impact of solitary confinement in the penal setting is to some extent analogous to those living alone for prolonged periods during lockdown. It is clearly not the same but bears our consideration. Even if only for a limited amount of time, it is reasonable to conclude that some of the mental challenges for people in pandemic lockdown will be similar, not least aspects of social death in living without physical social contact (even if social media mitigates for this) and dealing with 'dead time' when normal life and routines are put on hold. Guenther identifies how some prisoners in solitary confinement retain control of their environment through creating a schedule for their day. This is something we explore in relation to pandemic lockdown in Chapter 4.

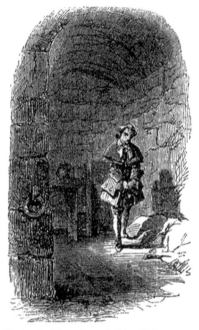

**Fig. 1.5. Solitary Confinement Engraving: John McLenan/
Public Domain.**

What Guenther identifies as the challenge in facing 'dead
time' during solitary confinement can also be thought of more
prosaically perhaps in terms of waiting. Patrick Rorke S.J., a
Catholic priest imprisoned under the Japanese during the
building of the Pakan Baroe railroad in Sumatra, summarised
the experience of confinement in this telling way:

> *P.O.W. life is summed up in this word: WAITING. To
> have to wait sustained by no real news, disappointed
> by the deceitfulness of rumours, on and on, week after
> week, month after month, for the great day.*

(Rorke, 1946, n.p.)

The capitalisation gets to the heart of the matter of the core challenge. Although we cannot possibly compare the pandemic lockdown with the awful conditions pertaining to the POW camps in Sumatra that Rorke and many others experienced during World War II, there is a similarity in the business of waiting, while confined, for news of an end to the situation. Not the 'great day' marking the end to hostilities but, in this case, that of freedom from lockdown.

For many, confinement during the pandemic will provoke thoughts of penal systems. Prisons and, in particular, notions of solitary confinement readily spring to mind. Large numbers of people will struggle to conceive previously homely environments in the same, familiar way. Now walls may feel as if they are closing in, doors holding them inside, viewpoints through windows limited, and time passing more slowly. They may be revisualising their dwellings as prisons or prison cells, be this alone or in groups. Similarly, many will be taking stock of what this all means to their mental health and well-being. Rather than divert our attention away from this sense of crossover between home and prison, it is perhaps here that we can best understand our emotional response to the new normal, take on board how the spaces we now occupy and the way we choose to live in them affect our bodies and minds and, indeed, our behaviours. We may also begin to consider how best to respond or adjust to the challenges ahead, especially dealing with cabin fever.

Confinement in prisons around the world is diverse but most share a similar restriction in freedom and space for those living in them. Prisoners or inmates are locked up in different kinds of small cells or holding areas. Some share cells, with overcrowding a feature of prison life worldwide. Others may be subject to spending prolonged periods of time on their own in solitary confinement. Cells may be visible from other cells or hidden from view. They may be empty or with limited furnishing or sanitation. Prisoners may be allowed some personal possessions or none at all. Materials that can be turned into weapons or ligatures will be outlawed. Heat, light, ventilation and noise levels may vary in different prison accommodations. Old buildings may be very noisy with hard surfaces intensifying the sounds. Modern institutions may be trauma-informed environments, more sensitive to reducing stressors, especially noise. The walls and floors may be dry or damp, rough or smooth, in various colours, with or without a window. Often the door to any cell will be heavily fortified and mostly metal as in the image below of the solitary confinement provision at the West Virginia State Penitentiary which operated from 1876 to 1995 (Fig. 1.6). Most prisons will have a routine for communication, washing, feeding, exercise and so on. This routine will be symbolised with particular sounds such as jangling keys, footfall, opening and closing of doors, conversation or bodily noises. These environments will also be marked by different smells and insect life.

In his book, *The Prison Community* (1940), Donald Clemmer highlighted the repetitive routines and monotony of prison life. This has changed little since then with ongoing concern about the penal milieu (Jordan, 2011; Sifunda et al., 2006). Such environments confine inmates with very restricted private space (Coyle, 2005) in an emotionally oppressive atmosphere, subject to overcrowding, high stress levels and trauma (Crewe, Hulley, & Wright, 2017; Jewkes, Jordan, Wright, & Bendelow, 2019).

DIVERSE LOCKDOWN

Beyond the penal system parameters of confinement, populations from nation to nation will be experiencing confinement resulting from pandemic lockdown in diverse ways, not least

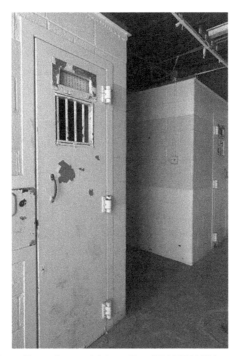

Source: https://www.loc.gov/pictures/item/2015632112/.

Fig. 1.6. Solitary Confinement Cells at the West Virginia State Penitentiary, a Retired, Gothic-Style Prison in Moundsville, West Virginia, that Operated from 1876 to 1995. No Known Restrictions on Publication.

because of differences in the kinds of accommodation or dwellings available to individuals or groups, in particular their spatial dimensions, occupancy numbers and density of these in rural or urban locations. In inner-city locations, especially among the poorest communities, dwellings may be very small, cramped and overcrowded with little or no access to green spaces. For example, a particular challenge in managing outbreaks of coronavirus came with high density, high rise accommodation. In Melbourne, Australia, authorities struggled with the 'explosive potential' of this challenge in nine sites (Visontay & Henriques-Gomes, 2020).

Beyond these built environment differences, individuals and households will be subject to diverse levels of economic, social and psychological stressors. Any of the following may exacerbate living conditions at this time: poverty, poor coping skills, limited access to heating, light, food and water, restricted social and cultural assets at home, or online and relational conflict. People will have different states of resiliency. While some individuals may easily bear isolation, others may succumb to despair, harming themselves or others. Similarly, families and groups may adjust and cope well with a long period of social distancing while others implode and fragment. We also need to bear in mind that lockdown for families will be very different depending on the number of children and adults, including vulnerable older relatives or those with underlying health conditions, sharing the physical space. In addition, the family dynamics during lockdown may be more complex and disrupted when parents or other adults have to leave or remain in the property to work. This may raise tensions when going out to work and returning potentially exposes family members to coronavirus infection or when working from home and engaged in demanding tasks requiring concentration and focus. In particular, people will face new soundscapes and potentially challenging noise levels, some of whom may be more prone to noise sensitivity and noise annoyance (Schreckenberg, Griefahn, & Meis, 2010; Shepherd, Welch, Dirks, & Mathews, 2010).

Gayer-Anderson et al. (2020) identify 'disproportionate' impacts of 'social isolation on disadvantaged, marginalised, and vulnerable populations in the context of pandemics and other public health crises' (p.1). The core impacts are increased mental health problems, inequalities in income, employment, access to food and discrimination. The latter has been particularly foregrounded during the pandemic following the killing

of George Floyd in the United States, with increased promi-
nence of the Black Lives Matter movement and protests globally, as well as concern about the disproportionate impact of
coronavirus on communities of colour. In addition, as noted
above, 'social restrictions that confine people to their homes for
extended periods increase risk of abuse and exploitation,
particularly among girls and women'. Complying with social
distancing measures is also 'most difficult for those on low
incomes, in insecure employment, and living in overcrowded
homes' (p. 5). Particularly badly affected are vulnerable populations who are healthcare workers, young people, those on
low incomes or with pre-existing conditions. Although there is
little data on other key, vulnerable individuals such as refugees
and the homeless, the impacts are likely to be similar.

ALTERED SOUNDSCAPES

The pandemic has changed our soundscapes in a number of
ways. Truax (1999a) defines a soundscape as 'an environment
of sound (or sonic environment) with emphasis on the way it is
perceived and understood by the individual, or by a society'
(n.p.). For those living in close quarters, particularly in restricted
accommodation, intrusive or interruptive noise may cause
profound irritation and impact on physical and mental health.
In such circumstances, individuals may be subject to the
unwanted, persistent noises of others with little respite. The
literature indicates the potential impact of noise, that is
unwanted, annoying, loud or interruptive sound (Truax,
1999a), on people's mental and physical health (e.g. Grebennikov & Wiggins, 2006; Hardoy et al., 2005; Honold, Beyer,
Lakes, & van der Meer, 2012; Leather, Beale, & Sullivan, 2003;
Miles, Coutts, & Mohamadi, 2012; Quehl & Basner, 2006;
Rocha, Pérez, Rodríguez-Sanz, Obiols, & Borrell, 2012;

Wallenius, 2004). Stansfeld and Matheson (2003) write that 'noise is more harmful to health in situations where several stressors interact … [leading to] chronic sympathetic arousal or states of helplessness' (pp. 253–254). The increased noise pollution of families in lockdown clearly has its own particular dangers, with other relational or financial stressors perhaps seeding the ground for various kinds of domestic abuse.

For those living alone but who previously had adult or child family members living with them the acoustic environment may be quite different and potentially challenging in terms of long periods of silence. For some that may be a relief while others may struggle with the intensification of solitude to the point of feeling acoustically deprived or cut off. Conversely, such individuals may be listening to music more and even turning up the volume to drown out the silence. In those households with several members, the imposition of noise, or unwanted sound, may lead to conflict and acoustic oppression as individuals seek peace and quiet, not least from incessant or intrusive TV, radio or conversation. What is not in doubt is that fulsome or depleted sonic environments will have different impacts on individuals and groups in their diverse dwellings. As such we can imagine a variety of responses to different challenges in our 'acoustic communities' (e.g. Schafer, 1994; Truax, 1999a, 1999b, 2001, 2002).

To illustrate this point, the first author PC found a number of sonic changes with positive and negative impacts on his emotions during the prolonged lockdown in the United Kingdom (which for him lasted 90 days). First, there was the perhaps expected challenge of dealing with long periods of relative silence that intensified the sense of aloneness and being cut off. Even frequent telephone calls or TV shows did not assuage this loss of one-to-one, in-person conversation. Perhaps one of the most profound sonic experiences of the pandemic lockdown is not so much noise but rather the absence of it. Importantly, we can begin to consider silence as offering two contrasting possibilities during the enforced lockdown. On the one hand, silence can prove deleterious in, as it clearly is in solitary confinement, bringing a 'rejection of the human personality' or, on the other hand, creating a meditative or sacred environment (Schafer, 1994). Second, the sonic rise of nature with bird song featured prominently. This was so evident that he happily began to take interest in the birds visiting his garden for the first time in his life, encouraging their presence by providing a feeder and water, and listening to and learning their calls. Truax (2001) describes listening as:

> *the crucial interface between the individual and the*
> *environment. It is also a set of sophisticated skills*
> *that appear to be deteriorating with the*
> *technologized urban environment, both because of*
> *noise exposure, which causes hearing loss and*
> *physiological stress, and because of the proliferation*
> *of low information, highly redundant, and basically*
> *uninteresting sounds, which do not encourage*
> *sensitive listening.*

(p. 15)

Brown, Rutherford, and Crawford (2015) underline the value of listening to natural sounds to improve mental health (something we pick up in the final chapter):

> *Sounds such as rain, a breeze, the sea, moving*
> *water and songbirds can calm and create a sense of*
> *wellbeing by triggering the release of endorphins, the*
> *body's natural opiates. Courtyards and landscaped*
> *gardens close to patient areas should include plants*
> *that encourage songbirds.*

(p. 1522)

Third, he found himself listening to music more and even setting up a solo disco with lights in the evenings. As with the sounds of nature, Brown et al. (2015) emphasised the calming, painkilling impact of music and its uses in countering depression, reducing blood pressure and so on. Fourth, a new routine of clapping, bashing saucepans or ringing bells from people's thresholds occurred on Thursday evenings for much of the official lockdown across the United Kingdom to show support for the National Health Service (NHS). This was a novel soundscape, or what Truax (1999a) calls a 'sound mark', specially regarded or unique to a community. Fifth, and less positively, and possibly like many other citizens, he grew irritated with or startled by sounds of racing car engines as some drivers exploited the empty streets at all hours or when delivery personnel no doubt under time pressures rapped or banged on the front door.

The pandemic, therefore, created a less familiar soundscape, one in which some sounds were lost and others added. In particular, for those unexpectedly in solitary lockdown and otherwise geared for social interaction the absence of the human voice would take its toll. Truax (2001) argues that the human voice is a key sound that represents the concept of 'self and relationships with others' and the environment. Without this, the kind of relational support and company voice brings is compromised. Monologue replaces dialogue. In an attempt to mitigate this loss, author PC began talking to himself on frequent occasions during lockdown. Quite aside from voice, other losses come with this isolation, such as the removal of sounds of movement or activities, even breathing, of others. As Garrioch (2003) notes, soundscapes give a 'feel' to places, making them familiar to us. It is clear from the experience of PC, that the lockdown separated him from his usual soundscape, that 'semiotic system, conveying news, helping people to locate themselves in time and in space, and making them part of an "auditory community"' (Garrioch, 2003, p. 5; see also Norman, 1996).

Of course, the impacts of changed soundscapes in the pandemic are not limited to people's dwellings. They extend to the eerily quiet, empty streets and loss of access to other familiar acoustic environments be they shops, schools, houses of worship or football stadiums. All such changes, at an acoustic level, can have an impact on how we view ourselves or our identity. Indeed, we may begin to wonder how the new unfamiliar or removed familiar sound symbols are constructing new identities, new senses of self and society (Bal, Crewe, & Spitzer, 1998), for better or worse. For example, if people are getting used to the more intense soundscape of nature, will they welcome a return to the noise of busy urban life? Will they be inspired to reduce car and air travel? What is not in doubt is that sounds are playing their part in the experience of the pandemic lockdown. In unfamiliar isolation, sounds can become a threat, a warning and stressor or offer comfort and reassurance. Sounds can spark different emotions. They are, as Schafer (1994) notes, primordial; they resonate with us, make us happy or make us jump out of our skins.

LOCKDOWN BENEFITS

At the same time, and perhaps counterintuitively, there appear to be some benefits emerging from the enforced lockdown such as enhanced relationships. For example, as much as China incurred increased divorce rates and relational conflict, it also witnessed strengthening connections with family and friends (Yi-Ling, 2020). Around 19% of couples surveyed in the United Kingdom reported enhanced relationships with their partners as opposed to around 10% stating a deterioration. A total 23% of parents reported improved relationships with their children as opposed to 10% who indicated a deterioration (Lancaster-James, 2020). Allington et al. (2020a) found that 60% of those surveyed had offered help to others and 47% had received help from others. People may also feel the impetus during lockdown to spend time through social media with older relatives who may well have had little attention previously or enhancing their connection with local communities and neighbours. In the era of negative news, these positive responses to the challenges of confinement suggest that cabin fever is not inevitable.

The perceived benefits from the shift to the use of social media during lockdown is perhaps unsurprising given earlier research. For example, a study conducted before the pandemic by Teo, Markwardt, and Hinton (2019) showed that older adults who use video chat, such as Skype, have a lower risk of developing depression. That said, at the other end of the life span, a study by Mallen, Day, and Green (2003) found undergraduate students communicating with other students that were unknown to them preferred face-to-face over Internet chat room conversations. The face-to-face group of participants in the study felt closer to and self-disclosed more during the interaction. Perhaps, once the pandemic is over, we will gain a stronger understanding of just how influential social media has been in mitigating the isolation resulting from the lockdown.

CABIN FEVER RISING

Despite some of the comforts of nature's sounds, or enhanced digital connectivity, the experience of prolonged confinement has proved extremely challenging for many. As time passed, during which young populations endured lockdown to save the lives of more vulnerable and older populations, the strain became more obvious. As nations continued to find their way in managing the spread of coronavirus while balancing the needs of the economy, many young people and families with children went 'stir crazy', engaging in risky public activities, not least street parties or raves, crowding parks and beaches. Even politically driven rallies or marches became prone to a complete lack of concern for the pandemic and its impacts. This recklessness in the face of the pandemic can be interpreted as a breaking out from the physical and psychological restrictions of lockdown. In effect, they evidenced a kind of cabin fever. This abandonment of caution, despite the warnings of national governments, extended to cases of premature social contact among sports people and their fans. Denied the drug of sport it seems both have been willing to forego human safety. Famously, Novak Djokovic led a tennis tournament in Serbia that did not follow social distancing rules, ending up with the star, among others, contracting the virus. Similarly, and on a much larger scale, fans of Liverpool Football Club celebrated their team winning the Premier League by gathering at close quarters in large numbers.

As the pandemic unfolded and multiple commentators discussed the psychological challenges of enforced confinement, a new, less dramatic term than cabin fever entered parlance that describes the public's inability to abide by imposed lockdown restrictions for long periods: lockdown fatigue. Not synonymous with the more extreme manifestations of cabin fever that accompanies the kind of isolation experienced wintering through in remote areas, this term pointed to disgruntlement with imposed rules in the context of good weather. The contrast between life indoors and the sunny outdoors became so stark that people felt compelled to venture out, travel into the countryside, the coast or other beauty spots, regardless of the risks.

Whether people have become simply tired of lockdown restrictions or more dramatically broken out of their isolation in more reckless ways underlining going 'stir crazy' after weeks or months confined in their homes, cabin fever has been compounded by or featured in a less visible way in the psychological torment among families and individuals. Bereavement has been blocked for many people unable to be with loved ones dying in intensive care units or nursing homes under strict quarantine. Family members have also struggled to even attend funerals. All this has intensified the deleterious isolation, mental health backdrop to the pandemic and the likelihood of poor psychological adjustment. This blocked bereavement has its parallel in cases where prison inmates have been prevented from access to normal grieving rituals or where the body of the deceased has remained lost or unavailable. There has also been serious concern and various initial reports about increased suicides around the world resulting from the pandemic and the social lockdown (e.g. Thakur & Jain, 2020; Thejesh, 2020; Vitelli, 2020) and among cruise ship workers struggling to deal with their rather extreme isolation away from access to ports (Bartlett, 2020; Greenfield & McCormick, 2020; Street, 2020).

The idea of a 'suicide pandemic' has been mooted, although at the time of writing this book, comprehensive data had not been made available. Yet this is very much expected. Mental health researchers such as Reger, Stanley, and Joiner (2020) have highlighted that the 'potential for adverse outcomes on suicide risk is high'. However, we must be cautious on the numbers as Carey (2020) summarises for the United States, where the impact of the pandemic on mortality has been large:

> *The mental health toll of the coronavirus pandemic is only beginning to show itself, and it is too early to predict the scale of the impact. … The ultimate marker of the virus's mental toll, some experts say, will show up in the nation's suicide rate, in this and coming years.*

We will also need to differentiate suicides relating to the pandemic and salient stressors such as isolation, financial insecurity and other pertinent losses or threats.

In the United Kingdom, the first peak of the outbreak coincided with the sunniest spring season on record (Met Office, 2020). This supported people in accessing their gardens and eventually parks and other rural and coastal landscapes as lockdown measures eased, bringing welcome relief from being trapped within the walls of their dwellings. Conversely, the glorious weather tantalised and taunted those without access to private gardens or green spaces, especially for millions of people with significant underlying health conditions shielding, that is, taking particular care to minimise contact with others. Yet immediate or eventual access to green spaces and the gradual easing of social distancing rules may well have mitigated cabin fever in the United Kingdom and other temperate zones. This is all the more reason to be concerned about the timing of any second or even third waves or peaks of the virus. These could easily coincide with extreme hot, cold or wet conditions that lend a new intensity to suffering confinement in any future lockdown. In particular, wintering out through a lockdown may yield new tales of woe not just for those susceptible to mental decline but also for those subject to domestic violence. The extreme versions of cabin fever may yet to be played out as the pandemic conspires with adverse meteorological and other conditions, not least social, economic and political ones. The global protests in the aftermath of the police killing of George Floyd in the United States showed that social unrest could add to the burden of threat from the pandemic with social distancing going into meltdown. It seems highly likely that enforced isolation will feature more rather than less for some time to come as nations struggle to contain the virus from successive outbreaks. As the response to the pandemic unfolds and with the distinct possibility of the spread of coronavirus being advanced in long winter flu seasons globally, with local or national lockdowns likely and mental health trauma continuing to exceed resources for support, cabin fever remains on the cards. By the time you pick up this book any number of new lockdowns may well have taken place with various manifestations and devastations of cabin fever.

In the next chapter (Chapter 2) we examine the origins and definitions of cabin fever and related folk terminology or idioms. In Chapter 3, we explore the social and cross-cultural history of this phenomenon in relation to life at close quarters at sea, on land, in the air and in space. In Chapter 4, we review the different antidotes to cabin fever, not least how isolation at home can provoke creative activities that mitigate and reduce its negative impacts. Whether we frame the greatest confinement in history as a kind of hibernation, suspended animation or perhaps more starkly as the kind of prolonged isolation found in penal systems there are aspects to the 'new normal' that defy passive suffering, trauma or irresolution. What has been particularly striking is the agency, ingenuity and creativity of individuals and communities while indoors.

2

A BRIEF HISTORY OF CABIN FEVER

ORIGINS

Early literary references to 'cabin fever' use the term to describe typhus, a contagious disease spread by lice (Fig. 2.1) that has blighted human populations since at least the fifteenth century CE, though medical historians have suggested it as a likely cause of the Plague of Athens in 430 BCE (Angelakis, Bechah, & Raoult, 2016; Raoult, Woodward, & Dumler, 2004; Urban, 1820). Before the Great Famine or *An Gorta Mór* (1845–1849) in Ireland many of the Irish poor, in rural locations, lived in single-room mud cabins or *an bothán* – according to the 1841 census 42% of Irish families occupied such dwellings (Robertson, 1879). These mud cabins became associated with the spread of typhus fever due to their confined and overcrowded space. Some cabins or *bothán scóir* were used by travelling farm labourers (McGarry, 2020), and this movement and the rural population's generosity in providing shelter to travellers, no doubt, increased infections. Indeed, as King (1927, p. 2644) indicates, the Irish people called typhus infection '"road fever," since it especially attacked wandering people'. He goes on:

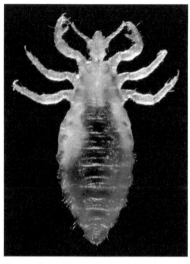

Credit: Janice Harney Carr, Center for Disease Control/Public domain
https://upload.wikimedia.org/wikipedia/commons/9/92/Body_lice.jpg.

Fig. 2.1. Typhus Lice.

*The inherent generosity of many natives would tend
to cause them to accept a wandering friend afflicted
with fever into their own house-holds, even though
overcrowded, rather than see him sent to an
institution. The tendency of large families to live in
overcrowded quarters, the sociable nature of the
people, causing them to exchange frequent and
prolonged visits with each other, and the custom of
observing wakes were factors bearing on the spread
of the disease.*

(King, 1927, p. 2646)

Long before and in the Great Famine, as McGarry (2020)
argues, '[c]abin dwellers did not stand a chance' in the face of

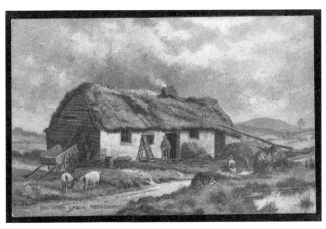

Fig. 2.2. An Irish Cabin, Roundwood.

infectious disease. Her description of such cabins underlines
the connection between such accommodation and the onset of
disease, not least fever (Fig. 2.2):

> *Cabins were basic, one-roomed and had few if no
> windows, a single lean-to door. There was a basic
> central hearth surrounded by stones, which was
> ventilated by a hole in the roof and used to cook
> food. Cabins were usually made of mud, sod, turf or
> scrap timber. Many were merely makeshift shelters,
> lean-tos with sods of earth for walls. Roofs were
> crudely thatched using heather or grass. They were
> draughty and damp and barely kept the weather out.
> There was obviously no electricity, running water or
> toilet in these dwellings. There was little or no
> furniture. Sleeping arrangements were pragmatic: the
> whole family, parents and children, slept together on
> the floor beside the fire. Cabin occupants had faces*

> *that were blackened by the fire smoke. Livestock, if*
> *any, shared these dwellings with humans. Directly*
> *outside the entrance to most cabins was a compost*
> *heap, known as a 'midden', containing household*
> *waste.*

Various scholars have studied the relationship between typhus fever and the cabins of labourers in Ireland during the Great Famine (e.g. Campbell, 1994; Derby, 2000; Kinealy & Moran, 2019). Kinealy & Moran (2019) quote a recollection of Henry Robinson about providing relief to those affected:

> *I remember going into one cabin where a widow was*
> *weeping piteously over her only son, whose body*
> *was lying under a sheet on the bed. He was her sole*
> *support, she said, and I took all particulars and*
> *assured her that I would recommend the maximum*
> *grant. Before leaving the cabin I went to the bed and*
> *gently lifted the corner of the sheet to look at the*
> *dead face. I was much taken aback when a bright*
> *blue eye met mine and regarded me with an*
> *expression of the deepest anxiety.*

> (p. 348)

With typhus outbreaks coinciding with food shortage, cabins came to be identified as synonymous with fever. After the Great Famine, three-roomed cottages replaced cabins as the accommodation of the rural poor. This was because cabins had low rental value and got in the way of grazing livestock, a more profitable use of land (McGarry, 2020). It is likely that the unattributed notion of 'cabin fever' emerged from this kind of context of small insanitary accommodation lending itself to infection in Ireland or elsewhere alongside other variant terms such as 'road fever' or 'famine fever' (Kinealy & Moran, 2019, p. 394). Lyons (1872, pp. 2–3) presents a great diversity of nomenclature in his treatise on relapsing or famine fever, not least typhus. In a study of the epidemiology of typhus fever in 1927, and without established 'separate statistics' for this malady, M.R. King wrote:

> *Since the beginning of authentic medical records typhus fever has held first place as a devastating disease among the inhabitants of Ireland, an unenviable reputation which the country has held until recent years. It is very probable that the plagues which accompanied the earliest civil wars [in the seventeenth century] were principally epidemic typhus.*

(King, 1927, pp. 2641–2642)

King notes the co-occurrence of substantial poverty and famine in

> *...an explosive outbreak of fever and a vast emigration which is probably without parallel in the history of Europe. The typhus epidemic that accompanied the potato famine was probably the worst that has ever visited the country.*

(King, 1927, p. 2664)

The Great Famine resulted in the great escape, with the emigration of 1.5 million Irish to North America (Constitutional Rights Foundation, 2010), swelling the numbers of Scotch-Irish already on the continent. Once there they played a key part in the pioneering migration and frontierism west in the nineteenth century (see Christensen, 1984), but not before introducing typhus to North America (see Baxter, 2009; Gelston & Jones, 1977) and being subject to various quarantine measures such as being held in 'fever sheds' in Canada (Gallagher, 1936). The latter were redolent of the earlier plague or pest-houses used in England back to the fourteenth century to quarantine infected people. Indeed, some pest-houses, such as that at Deddington in Oxfordshire (see Robinson, 1980), were little more than simple, single-storey dwellings resembling the Irish mud huts or cabins. Although this fact may lend itself to the genealogy of 'cabin fever', there is little historical evidence of an explicit link between these pest-houses and the folk term. It is perhaps more likely that the erstwhile physical fever or typhus-related term 'cabin fever' came into use first after the Irish emigrants introduced the disease to North America and then in describing the feverish psychological affliction from prolonged confinement in makeshift, frontier cabin dwellings, with which they became closely associated. This link is all the more compelling when we note that while the introduction of log cabins in the United States had been by Swedes settling in Delaware in the seventeenth century, as Morrison (1987) writes:

> *English colonists were reluctant to use the log cabin for dwelling purposes, even in the eighteenth-century, and it was the Scotch-Irish who did most to popularise its use. Coming from a land of inferior housing conditions, they found it highly practical and satisfactory. Penetrating to the frontier of Maine and New Hampshire, pushing westward across the Alleghenies and southward into Virginia and North Carolina, the Scotch-Irish made the log cabin a symbol of the American pioneer. The form became common by the mid-eighteenth century, and the name 'log cabin' in its modern sense was first used in an Irish community in the valley of Virginia in 1770.*

(p. 13)

Importantly, knowledge about infectious disease was only developing robustly towards the end of the nineteenth century and prior to this, symptoms such as stupor and delirium may easily have been attributed to either the physical disease of typhus or psychological affliction due to prolonged confinement. This may explain the elision of the two different kinds of health challenge over time and, with improved housing, sanitation, and abatement of infectious disease, the eventual adoption of the term 'cabin fever' as referring to a folk or culture-bound psychological syndrome that became apparent in the pioneering frontierism comprising wintering in remote, small makeshift cabins in which Irish immigrants played a key part, for example, moving beyond city life in New York, Boston and Chicago, as labourers laying down new railroads or trying to make their fortune joining the search for gold (Emmons, 2010; O'Laughlin, 2007).

Both the physical and psychological frames of 'cabin fever' are predicated on the notion of the 'cabin', a term for a simple one-storey dwelling, as is the case with the Irish mud huts or other temporary or hastily built wooden dwellings. Log-built cabins have a history stretching back to the Bronze Age in Northern and Eastern Europe, long before their use in the United States and North America more broadly (Belonsky, 2017; Kniffen & Glassie, 1966). Favoured as a simple-to-construct dwelling in remote but tree-rich areas of the world, the log cabin is an iconic architecture that connotes austerity, humility and independence. It also connotes isolation or retreat from society. These simple dwellings could be makeshift, without the use of nails or more elaborate design, convenient to hunting, pioneer and frontier settlement in remote locations or for other immediate or timely migrations, as in the gold rushes of the early American West (Fig. 2.3).

The precise origin and circulation of the term 'cabin fever' is unclear. While there is no extant reference to 'cabin fever'

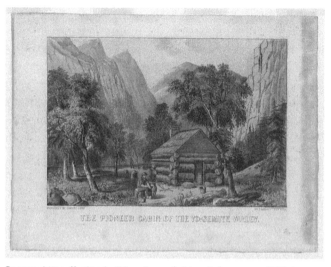

**Fig. 2.3. Pioneer Cabin Yosemite Valley. Graphic Arts/
Public Domain [Higher Resolution Available].**

per se, to our knowledge, in Irish accounts of typhus or other
contagious outbreaks such as cholera at the time, there was
clear, expressed concern about the role that crowded cabins
played in spreading infections in Ireland. The majority of Irish
people emigrating to America in and around the Great Famine
were from the poor, labouring classes, so very well aware of
the link between poverty, poor housing, such as cabins, and
the onset of typhus fever and death. It is likely that this
knowledge remained a cultural reference point for them connecting cabin spaces with symptoms of fever (regardless of
physical or psychological aetiology). The earliest published
reference to the term, supporting this hypothesis, appears to
be in 1820, associating it with typhus and the Irish context:

> *The certain consequence is the low typhus or cabin fever, which at all times, and at this present moment, exists in Ireland to a degree, that in any other country would create a serious alarm.*
>
> (Urban, 1820, p. 139)

While Andrew Belonsky (2018) mistakenly attributes coining of the term to B.M. Bowers, the earliest references to 'cabin fever' in newspaper archives are reviews of her novel, *Cabin Fever* (1918). It is noteworthy that even then, some 100 years after the reference by Sylvanus Urban (pseudonym of Edward Cave) in *The Gentleman's Magazine*, a number of American publications feel it necessary to define the term in quotations, suggesting an unfamiliarity with it (e.g., Richmond Times-Dispatch, 1918, p. 4). A review in New York City's *The Sun* (The Sun, 1918, p. 10) defined the term as being synonymous with 'wanderlust', which may further hint at the earlier, albeit obfuscated connection with concerns about the spread of typhus by travellers in Ireland as much as those migrating to new frontiers in the United States. Wanderlust connotes a strong desire, impulse or irresistible urge to escape or be free of a fixed or confining place, to move on, to experience a changed scene and not remain in one spot. Merriam-Webster (n.d.) defines it as a 'strong longing for or impulse toward wandering' and provides its German roots as follows:

> *For my part,* writes Robert Louis Stevenson in Travels with a Donkey, *'I travel not to go anywhere, but to go. I travel for travel's sake. The great affair is to move.' Sounds like a case of wanderlust if we ever heard one. Those with 'wanderlust' don't necessarily need to go anywhere in particular; they just don't care to stay in one spot. The etymology of* wanderlust

is a very simple one that you can probably figure out
yourself. 'Wanderlust' is lust (or 'desire') for
wandering. The word comes from German, in which
wandern *means 'to wander,' and* Lust *means 'desire.'*

The first paragraph of B.M. Bower's *Cabin Fever* (1918)
provides an interesting and diverse encapsulation of the
affliction in this period:

THERE is a certain malady of the mind induced by
too much of one thing. Just as the body fed too long
upon meat becomes a prey to that horrid disease
called scurvy, so the mind fed too long upon
monotony succumbs to the insidious mental ailment
which the West calls "cabin fever." True, it parades
under different names, according to circumstances
and caste. You may be afflicted in a palace and call it
ennui, and it may drive you to commit peccadillos
and indiscretions of various sorts. You may be
attacked in a middle-class apartment house, and call
it various names, and it may drive you to cafe life and
affinities and alimony. You may have it wherever you
are shunted into a backwater of life, and lose the
sense of being borne along in the full current of
progress. Be sure that it will make you abnormally
sensitive to little things; irritable where once you
were amiable; glum where once you went whistling
about your work and your play. It is the crystallizer
of character, the acid test of friendship, the final seal
set upon enmity. It will betray your little, hidden
weaknesses, cut and polish your undiscovered
virtues, reveal you in all your glory or your vileness
to your companions in exile—if so be you have any.

There will be historically bound differences in the phenomenon of cabin fever, not least perspectives on its intensity. How might cabin fever then be best defined? What might we learn relevant to its symptoms from prison literature and research on solitary confinement? Also, cases of cabin fever are not limited to land environments but also occur at sea, in the air and in space. We will now examine the ways that cabin fever has been defined and researched in relation to these different places, with reference to representations of the condition in cultural production, especially literature, memoir and reportage which offer imaginative access to the condition.

DEFINITIONS

We can define a cabin as a restricted compartment or dwelling. As a compartment we may include spaces for crew, drivers, pilots, passengers or cargo on a variety of vehicles (e.g., ships, boats, submarines, spacecraft, planes, trains, buses, lorries, vans, taxis). As outlined above, in architecture, a cabin typically denotes a small, simple one-storey dwelling or hut (from L. *capanna*), often made of wood (e.g., a log cabin).

The word fever typically refers to a person having an abnormally high or pyrexial body temperature with symptoms of headache, shivering and even delirium. We think perhaps of typhus, malaria or influenza. The etymological root is in burn, heat, fire, ashes and summer. But it also refers to a state of nervous excitement. This notion may have come from the Sanskrit *bhur*, meaning to be restless (Online Etymology Dictionary, n.d.).

Both the separate notions of 'cabin' and 'fever' combine in 'cabin fever' which is not a medically defined condition but a 'folk belief' (Christensen, 1984) or

> *...folk term ... commonly understood to refer to some combination of irritability, moodiness, boredom, depression, or feeling of dissatisfaction in response to confinement, bad weather, routine, isolation, or lack of stimulation.*
>
> (Rosenblatt, Anderson, & Johnson, 1984, p. 44)

This can afflict an individual or group experiencing prolonged isolation on land, at sea, in the air and in space. The noun cabin fever is defined in the Collins English Dictionary (n.d., Definition 2) as an 'acute depression resulting from being isolated or sharing cramped quarters in the wilderness, esp during the long northern winter'. The Cambridge Dictionary (n.d., Definition 1) defines it more generally as 'the feeling of being angry and bored because you have been inside for too long'. We may simplify such definitions to think of cabin fever as a popular notion applied to mental discomfort resulting from being in confined isolation for long periods.

While submariners, astronauts, miners or potholers tend to have high tolerance for confined isolation and may largely be able to manage any fear or anxiety, many of us may experience some discomfort or unease in such environments (Kinderman, 2016). For others, this discomfort can be particularly acute and feature in serious, partly overlapping phobias or anxiety disorders. Such individuals may fear open or public places (agoraphobia – literally 'fear of the marketplace') and enclosed spaces (claustrophobia). They may also experience panic in such environments. Curiously, those with agoraphobia will also avoid enclosed spaces such as elevators, crowded spaces, cars, buses and planes for fear of being embarrassed, unable to escape or get help. Such individuals can often become housebound. The main feature that differentiates the two conditions, given that both can happen in crowded or enclosed spaces, is that people with claustrophobia will not feel anxiety in an open space (Gelder, Adreasen, Lopez-Ibor, & Geddes, 2009; Renzoni, 2020).

There have been a number of studies on the psychological and social impact of the experience of isolation and cabin fever on land, at sea, in the air and in space. The popular syndrome of cabin fever has also featured in literature and various other cultural accounts, not least those relating to medicine and illness. In this chapter, the aim is not to totalise information about these but to provide an entry point to the topic of cabin fever in different places or circumstances, in particular in fiction and memoir.

Cabin fever features in the work of various writers who have experienced voluntary and enforced confinement and this chapter, in part, explores the curious contrast between isolation as affliction and as a spur to creativity. Many writers, philosophers and other creatives as diverse as Henry David Thoreau, Walt Whitman, Emily Dickinson, Bernard Shaw, D.H. Lawrence, Dylan Thomas and Ludwig Wittgenstein sought their muse by taking to cabins or sheds rather like hermits and mystics did before them for spiritual enlightenment in caves and huts. Henry David Thoreau, for example, described small dwelling experiences in his book *Walden* (1854), championing the simple life in natural surroundings. Tom Montgomery-Fate, in his book *Cabin Fever* (2011), which is a homage to Thoreau, explores both the solitude and the challenge of being lonely in a contemporary cabin in the woods. But his reflection offers more of a nature-infused counter to modern life than dealing head on with the darker and more desperate side of isolation in remote natural environments. For example, in her travel memoir *Stir Crazy in Kazakhstan* (2015), Katy Warner wrote about the mental challenges of living in an isolated farmhouse on the borders of Kazakhstan, Russia and China. In all, many works of fiction, memoir and poetry have flagged up that small spaces can be both havens and prisons. At their best confined dwellings can offer reassuring and meditative life-styles. At their worst they can provoke mental collapse and even suicide.

One aspect of enforced isolation that has been identified as a key factor in psychological difficulty is *ennui*, that is, a state of boredom or monotony. Since the film *Groundhog Day* (1993) starring Bill Murray, the term 'Groundhog Day' has entered general parlance, connoting boring, monotonous or repetitive experiences – something that many of those in lockdown will recognise. The mental challenge of boredom is neatly apparent in the title of a recent book by James Danckert and John D. Eastwood, *Out of My Skull: The Psychology of Boredom* (2020). Although the authors rightly outline the capacity for boredom to inspire creativity, they also warn that this state bedevils those without intrinsic motivation or with poor impulse control; those with narcissistic or hostile per-sonalities; and people who are subject to addiction. As such, boredom's 'spur to creativity' is countered by the darker likelihood of excessive consumption of social media and heightened hostility. One wonders whether the extreme boredom of social austerity and confinement will bring esca-lating social and political tumult and division beyond the hidden tragedy of domestic violence. Will intense, widespread boredom prove a revolutionary force? How devastating can cabin fever be on land, at sea, in the air and in space?

3

CABIN FEVER CASES

In this chapter, we explore cases of cabin fever on land, at sea, in the air and in space, starting with land, as this is where the term 'cabin fever' and other congruent culture-bound or folk syndromes emanate. Where relevant we will extend beyond research evidence to discuss illuminatory literature, memoir or reportage representing the kinds of experience that may occur in these dimensions. As we will see, cabin fever can lead to some extreme behaviours.

ON LAND

Various scholars have noted the mental health challenges of remote areas of Canada, such as the Yukon (Atcheson, 1972; Kehoe & Abbott, 1975). In small accommodation such as cabins or other simple dwellings this phenomenon is deemed as more likely to occur, but not exclusively, in winter months when outside environments may prove inaccessible. A person subject to cabin fever may suffer from sleeplessness (insomnia) or sleepfulness (hypersomnia). They may even develop paranoia and difficulty in rational decision-making. At its extreme, people may feel compelled to escape their spatial restrictions or limited routines, regardless of external conditions or the cost to themselves or others. An overwhelming panic can set in and undermine normal behaviour. Cabin fever may also lead to self- and other-directed violence, including suicide.

Prairie fever or madness is another 'folk term', alternate idiom or even synonymous expression related to 'cabin fever' and being 'stir crazy'. It too indicates symptoms arising from prolonged confinement (Pagnamenta, 2012; Underwood, 1985). Similar to 'cabin fever' it refers to the particular restrictions of being isolated and cooped up in harsh weather in remote areas. Such social austerity occurred, for example, in migration to the Canadian prairies, in particular, the Great Plains, in the nineteenth century. Prairies are best described as unremitting, flat grasslands. Symptoms experienced bear a close resemblance to those marking cabin fever, notably depression, cognitive disturbance, violence, suicide and withdrawal. Whilst the term 'prairie fever' is closely aligned with 'cabin fever' and 'stir crazy', it differs in placing an emphasis on isolation experienced by living in a vast, flat open space over the actual place of confinement, that is a cabin or prison. That said, all these terms point to extreme social dislocation resulting from highly restricted or compromised access to company. Whether in cabins and larger farm homesteads on the open plains, tucked in some remote, frontier woodland, in a makeshift hut in polar conditions, in restricted penal environments or in prolonged lockdown in urban or rural places, these terms coalesce in the mental challenge of isolation.

The notion of 'frontier' is indicative of new, undeveloped, remote areas of land which are explored and exploited for development, initially by pioneers, sometimes compromising the rights and freedoms of native inhabitants. In conceiving of the exploration of frontiers many people will have in mind the

United States as a key case, as its population stretched northwards and westwards. Various early and more recent commentators have explored the nature of the frontier (Cromartie, Nulph, Hart, & Dobis, 2013; Nobles, 1997; Turner, 1893, 1921). In his early overview of three 'waves' to the American frontier between the seventeenth and nineteenth centuries, Turner (1893) places the log cabin as the chief dwelling of pioneers:

> *He builds his cabin, gathers around him a few other families of similar tastes and habits, and occupies till the range is somewhat subdued, and hunting a little precarious, or, which is more frequently the case, till the neighbors crowd around, roads, bridges, and fields annoy him, and he lacks elbow room.*
>
> (n.p.)

Cromartie et al. (2013) summarise a common understanding of frontier in this territory at least as denoting 'relatively remote and sparsely settled' areas to be 'found largely but not exclusively in the Great Plains and Intermountain West' (p. 149). They point out the mixed benefits of the 'remoteness' of frontier land or hinterlands where access to beautiful landscapes comes with economic and social challenges and potentially negative impacts on well-being. In his book, *Miles from Nowhere* (1993), Dayton Duncan captures the freedoms and limitations of contemporary life on the edge of authority and mainstream. Again, for those choosing this way of life, taking pride in being self-reliant is, as Duncan indicates, often accompanied by the threat of dullness, boredom, depleted resources, alcohol issues and a propensity to violence.

Another culture-bound syndrome that, given its arctic or polar provenance, bears resemblance to cabin fever is Alaskan madness or *pibloktoq*. *Pibloktoq* is described as a form of 'arctic hysteria' among the Inuit (Foulks, 1972; Gussow, 1985; Landy, 1985). The entry in DSM-IV-TR (American Psychiatric Association, 2000, p. 901) for the syndrome is as follows:

> *An abrupt dissociative episode accompanied by extreme excitement of up to 30 minutes' duration and frequently followed by convulsive seizures and coma lasting up to 12 hours. This is observed primarily in arctic and subarctic Eskimo communities, although regional variations in name exist. The individual may be withdrawn or mildly irritable for a period of hours or days before the attack and will typically report complete amnesia for the attack. During the attack, the individual may tear off his or her clothing, break furniture, shout obscenities, eat feces, flee from protective shelters, or perform other irrational or dangerous acts.*

The updated version of DSM (DSM-5)[2] describes dissociative disorders as 'characterized by a disruption of and/or discontinuity in the normal integration of consciousness, memory, identity, emotion, perception, body representation, motor control, and behavior' (American Psychiatric Association, 2013, p. 291). In this revised manual, culture-bound syndromes appear under a new category, Cultural Concepts of Distress, but *pibloktoq* is no longer included. Interestingly, isolation is only mentioned 29 times, boredom has only 8 entries, and loneliness features on a measly 7 occasions across the entire manual. Curiously, there are only singular references to confinement and prison conditions as triggering acute dissociative states (American Psychiatric Association, 2013, p. 295). It is as if isolation, loneliness, confinement, prison conditions and boredom, all key aspects or drivers to the experience of cabin fever or going 'stir crazy', are barely worth mentioning in relation to mental health. Should we anticipate this will feature more prominently in a post-pandemic DSM-6 manual of psychiatric disorders?

Dick (1995) provides one of the most comprehensive overviews of the difficult-to-explain condition of *pibloktoq*. Among those who have considered the syndrome environmentally determined, the early Canadian ethnologist Diamond Jenness in his book, *The People of the Twilight* (1928), maintained that the condition was provoked by the loneliness and silence incurred in the region during dark winters. Another plausible syndrome considered in ethnopsychiatry that arguably resembles *pibloktoq* is *menerik*, noted to afflict remote Yakut, Yukaghir and Evenk communities in Siberia and also considered to relate to the monotony of life in this region (Sidorov & Davydov, 1992).

There is likely to be a crossover or relatedness between weather-determined cabin fever (i.e., trapped due to bad weather) and seasonal affective disorder (SAD) – afflicting people in cold, northern regions with low daylight hours. These are not *necessarily* connected however. Cabin fever is related to prolonged or extreme isolation, typically in restricted spaces. SAD (see Wirz-Justice, 2018) is not caused by or dependent on such isolation. That said, a person may be subject to the development of SAD due to a lack of sunlight as well as enduring enforced isolation resulting in cabin fever. Furthermore, SAD may be the more medically recognised correlate alongside claustrophobia of cabin fever, which, as a folk or culture-bound syndrome, falls outside a clinical frame. We also have to remember that the experience of isolation of the intense kind referred to in cabin fever can occur in a variety of dwellings and environments. Either way, the experience will result from a perception of enforced or restricted isolation with an inaccessible or threatening external environment. This restriction may result from the actions of others, as in imprisonment, making the outside world unavailable due to environments of extreme weather and other potentially harmful external conditions such as in air or space flight, a psychologically challenging wilderness, or, as in the case of this book, a pandemic. In the latter, the external environment could be diversely urban or rural, again with various additional stressors, for example, political, social and economic turmoil, lack of key resources, or many other factors such as intrusive noise levels or unnerving silence.

Quite aside from a more familiar view of cabin fever in terms of the provocation of confinement to small dwellings in adverse conditions, or solitary confinement in penal systems, we may wish to extend the compass to a much more everyday phenomenon: driving vehicles. Although road rage is invariably aligned with the driver's aloofness from danger and their right to the road, surrounded by the skin of the vehicle they are held within, it is worth considering how confinement in this context may be influencing driver emotion. Sansone and Sansone (2010) define 'road rage' as encompassing

> *...a variety of aggressive behaviors by the driver of a motor vehicle, which seem well beyond the perceived offence committed by the victim. These behaviors range from shouting, screaming, and yelling at another driver to using a weapon, including the vehicle, to incite damage to the victim or the victim's vehicle.*

> (p. 14)

They identify contributory environmental variables, such as 'crowded roads and high levels of traffic density; psychological factors, such as displaced anger, illogical attributions, and high life stress; and bona fide psychiatric disorders' (p. 16). Of interest here is the whole business of crowding and

density which we may consider as a mobile, dynamic intensification of confinement for motorists sequestered in the
vehicle's cabin. Perhaps future research might focus on in-
vehicle space limitations and perceptions of external space
restriction as a contributory factor, as claustrophobic. In other
words, maybe we should view road rage as an everyday
occurrence of cabin fever. To date, this aspect and potential
for cabin fever as contributory to road rage has not been
researched.

Cabins of one kind or another have featured in numerous
works of fiction, most memorably perhaps in Harriet Beecher
Stowe's melodramatic anti-slavery novel *Uncle Tom's Cabin;
or, Life Among the Lowly* (1852) which inadvertently
advanced negative stereotypes of black people:

> *The cabin of Uncle Tom was a small log building,
> close adjoining to 'the house,' as the negro* par
> excellence *designates his master's dwelling. In front
> of it had a neat garden-patch, where, every summer,
> strawberries, raspberries, and a variety of fruits and
> vegetables, flourished under careful tending. The
> whole front of it was covered by a large scarlet
> begonia and a native multiflora rose, which,
> entwisting and interlacing, left scarce a vestige of the
> brought logs to be seen.*

This near-idyll is reversed when Tom, a slave, is sold on
from the relatively 'benevolent' estate of Kentucky farmer
Arthur Shelby to a more violent and abusive plantation in
Louisiana, owned by Simon Legree:

> *Tom rose, disconsolate, and stumbled into the cabin
> that had been allotted to him. The floor was already
> strewn with weary sleepers, and the foul air of the
> place almost repelled him; but the heavy night-dews*

were chill, and his limbs weary, and, wrapping about
him a tattered blanket, which formed his only bed-
clothing, he stretched himself in the straw and fell
asleep.

Despite Tom's change in fortunes, the cabin, as described
by Stowe, remained the dwelling of the lowly, the poor and
the dispossessed.

There have also been fictional works that draw on or deal
substantively with the theme of cabin fever. For example,
Fyodor Dosteovsky creates a claustrophobic atmosphere in his
philosophical novella *Notes from Underground* (1864). In this
story, the narrator inhabits a dark crawl space under the
floorboards in which he battles inertia, extreme boredom or
ennui. The isolation and confinement is intensified through the
symbolism of a stone wall blocking freedom. In his later novel
Crime and Punishment (1866), Dostocvsky revisits this theme
when the main character Raskolnikov commits murder for a
high ideal before struggling with a punishing, entrapping
conscience. Raskolnikov's living conditions are pitched as a
maddening confinement, one that even extends to the street
and eventually to becoming psychologically cooped up in a
guilty mind following his crime. With personal experience of
confinement while serving hard labour in Siberia for sedition,
or later of being holed up, heavily in debt, in a small hotel
room in Weisbaden, Germany (see Magarshack, 1996, p. 9),
Dostoevsky has his character in similar straits and 'stifling'
mental despair on the opening pages of the novel. The whole
scene conveys a ubiquitous mood of cabin fever within and
without:

On a very hot evening at the beginning of July a
young man left his little room at the top of a house in
Carpenter Lane, went out into the street, and, as

*though unable to make up his mind, walked slowly in
the direction of Kokushkin Bridge.*

*He was lucky to avoid a meeting with his landlady on
the stairs. His little room under the very roof of a tall
five-storey building was more like a cupboard than a
living-room. … He was up to the neck in debt to his
landlady and was afraid of meeting her.*

*It was not as though he were a coward by nature or
easily intimidated. Quite the contrary. But for some
time past he has been in an irritable and overstrung
state which was like hypochondria. He had been so
absorbed in himself and had led so cloistered a life
that he was afraid of meeting anybody. …*

*It was terribly hot in the street, and the stifling air,
the crowds of people, the heaps of mortar
everywhere, the scaffolding, and the bricks, the dust
and that peculiar summer stench which is so familiar
to everyone who lives in Petersburg and cannot
afford to rent a cottage in the country - all that had a
most unfortunate effect on the young man's already
overwrought nerves.*

(Dostoevsky, 1866 [Trans. 1996], pp. 19–20)

The cramped, claustrophobic conditions of Raskolnikov's
room are flagged up time and again, not least as resembling a
ship's cabin:

*He woke up late next morning after a disturbed
night. His sleep had not refreshed him. He woke up
feeling ill-humoured, irritable, and cross, and he
looked around his little room with hatred. It was a
tiny cubicle, about six feet in length, which looked
most miserable with its dusty, yellowish paper*

*peeling off the walls everywhere. It was, besides, so
low that even a man only a little above average
height felt ill at ease in it, fearing all the time that he
might knock his head against the ceiling.*

(p. 45)

And later in the novel:

*But at that moment the door was again flung open
and, stooping a little, because he was very tall,
Razumikhin came into the room.*

*'What a ship's cabin!' he cried, entering. 'Always
knock my head against the door. And they call it a
room!..'*

(p. 137)

We noted earlier the explicit treatment of the impact of
restricted confinement in B.M. Bower's (1918) *Cabin Fever:
A Novel*. Another novel along these lines is Willa Cather's
O Pioneers! (1913), a story about the prairie madness of
Nebraskan homesteaders in the late nineteenth century. The
psychological challenge for the homesteaders lies with both
the isolation and loneliness of their farmland, not least
through the winters, and in the face of an overwhelming,
surrounding wild wasteland. In the novel, Ivar becomes
mentally unstable in his remote farmstead and is only saved
from the lunatic asylum by being taken in as a servant to the
main character, Alexandra. Another character, Frank, ends up
as an extremely irritable, hard-drinking man who kills his wife
and her lover, Alexandra's younger brother, Emil. This theme
of mental challenge from settlement in remote areas features
in other works such as James Mitchener's *Centennial* (1976),
set in the Colorado plains, and, quite recently, Michael

F. Parker's *Prairie Fever* (2019) which tells the story of two sisters isolated on the grasslands of Oklahoma.

Such stories of the wilderness and the threat of isolation and descent into madness offer an imaginative window on the folk syndrome of cabin or prairie fever. Other literature explores isolation on desert islands, a popular theme in literature. For example, there is Daniel Defoe's *The Life and Strange Surprizing Adventures of Robinson Crusoe* (1719), Johann David Wyss's *The Swiss Family Robinson* (1812) and William Golding's *Lord of the Flies* (1954). A further literary angle on isolation comes with fiction about extreme kinds of incarceration as in Stefan Zweig's treatment of Dr B., mentally scarred by confinement under the Nazis in his novella *Chess* (1941), Room 101, a torture chamber, in George Orwell's *Nineteen Eighty-Four: A Novel* (1949), or Henri Charriére's *Papillon* (1969) about incarceration and escape from an isolated French penal colony. In Zweig's *Chess*, Dr B recounts his seclusion as a special case, being softened up for interrogation in a private hotel rather than concentration camp:

> *For the pressure they intended to exert, to get the "material" they needed out of us, was to operate more subtly than through crude violence and physical torture: the method was the most exquisitely refined isolation. Nothing was done to us – we were simply placed in a complete void, and everyone knows that nothing on earth exerts such pressure on the human soul as a void. Solitary confinement in a complete vacuum, a room hermetically cut off from the outside world, was intended to create pressure not from without, through violence and the cold, but from within, and to open our lips in the end.*
>
> (Zweig, 1941 [Trans. 2017], p. 40)

Using repetition to great effect, Zweig captures the pain of the social void, the interminable waiting that Patrick Rorke SJ identified in POW camps, isolated 'like a diver under a glass dome in the black ocean of this silence':

> *You kept waiting for something from morning to evening, and nothing happened. You waited again, and yet again. Nothing happened. You waited, waited, waited, you thought, you thought, you thought until your head was aching. Nothing happened. You were left alone. Alone. Alone.*
>
> (Zweig, 1941 [Trans. 2017], p. 41)

Literature dealing with social isolation in urban settings, deteriorating mentally under what Zweig calls the 'terrible same' (p. 41) which eventually results in 'brain fever' (p. 68), seems especially pertinent to our concern with confinement during the pandemic. Another earlier and important fiction in this regard is *The Yellow Wallpaper* (1892) by Charlotte Perkins Gilman which powerfully evokes not just confinement of a woman in a physical sense but also psychologically in a way that is familiar to us as domestic violence. The narrator is effectively trapped by her doctor husband who gaslights her, manipulates and controls her identity and restricts her freedom. Much more recently, J.G. Ballard's novels *Concrete Island* (1974) and *High Rise* (1975) explore the physical and mental dangers of social isolation, while Elizabeth Jolley's novel *Cabin Fever* (1991) charts the main character Vera's reflections on the isolation and escape that relationships can bring while confined to a small hotel room in New York.

The isolation of groups of people, of course, has played out in various literature representing contagion, pestilence and quarantine. Perhaps one of the most harrowing accounts is Daniel Defoe's *A Journal of the Plague Year* (1722) which details the 1665 'great visitation' in London. His description of the shutting up of infected and non-infected family members, the 'distemper' of those in delirium, the impact on social contact and even the comforts of marking the death of individuals is highly pertinent to households during the coronavirus lockdown. In particular, we gain a sense of 'cabin fever' resulting from the enforced quarantine in the limited spaces of dwellings.

First, people experienced intense anxiety being incarcerated and under threat of infection:

> *[I]t was generally in such houses that we heard the most dismal shrieks and outcries of the poor people, terrified and even frighted to death by the sight of the condition of their dearest relations, and by the terror of being imprisoned as they were.*

(Defoe, 1722, n.p.)

Second, the confinement brought the distress of limited social interaction (Fig. 3.1):

> *They had no way to converse with any of their friends but out at their windows, where they would make such piteous lamentations as often moved the hearts of those they talked with, and of others who, passing by, heard their story; and as those complaints oftentimes reproached the severity, and sometimes the insolence, of the watchmen placed at their doors.*

(n.p.)

Third, the fear and restlessness in confinement erupted in violence:

> *[M]any people perished in these miserable confinements which, 'tis reasonable to believe, would*

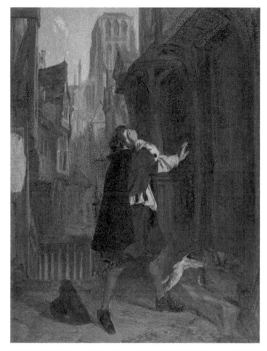

**Fig. 3.1. 'An Incident in the Great Plague of London' by
Alexander Christie**

*not have been distempered if that had had liberty,
though the plague was in the house; at which the
people were very clamorous and uneasy at first, and
several violences were committed and injuries offered
to the men who were set to watch the houses so shut
up; also several people broke out by force in many
places.*

(n.p.)

Fourth, as we noted earlier, there is a crossover and blurring between the psychological distress and resultant extreme behaviours we think of as cabin fever and physical symptoms of infection:

> *A house in Whitechapel was shut up for the sake of one infected maid, who had only spots, not the tokens come out upon her, and recovered: yet these people obtained no liberty to stir, neither for air or exercise, forty days. Want of breath, fear, anger, vexation, and all the other gifts attending such an injurious treatment cast the mistress into a fever, and visitors came into the house and said it was the plague, though the physicians declared it was not. However, the family were obliged to begin their quarantine anew on the report of the visitors or examiner, though their former quarantine wanted but a few days of being finished. This oppressed them so with anger and grief, and, as before, straitened them also so much to room, and for want of breathing and free air, that most of the family fell sick.*

(n.p.)

Alongside a growing sense of injustice in being subject to claustrophobic lockdown, and disappointment in having to repeat it, which mirror contexts in the current pandemic, those confined under the quarantine Defoe describes also suffered blocked grief as the sick of the household were 'not permitted to die at large' or have their passing marked in the normal way.

As noted in Crawford, Greenwood, Bates, and Memel (2020b), various 'outbreak novels' in the nineteenth century included the theme of the Plague and other epidemics, such as Elizabeth Gaskell's *Ruth* (1853), Harriet Martineau's *Sickness and Health of the People* (1853) and George Eliot's *Romola* (1863). In the twentieth century, a wide array of fiction has extended the theme of contagion in many different ways, such as Katherine Anne Porter's *Pale Horse, Pale Rider* (1939), Albert Camus's *The Plague* (1947), Michael Crichton's *The Andromeda Strain* (1969), John Christopher's *Empty World* (1977), Stephen King's *The Stand* (1978), Gabriel García Márquez's *Love in the Time of Cholera* (1985), Mario Bellatin's *Beauty Salon* (1994), Margaret Atwood's *Oryx and Crake* (2002), José Saramago's *Blindness* (2013) and St. John Mandel's *Station Eleven* (2014).

In Saramago's *Blindness*, for example, an epidemic causing blindness leads the authorities to confine victims in an empty mental hospital where they are exploited and assaulted by a criminal element. This nightmarish frame, not least of violence towards women, underlines the mental affliction of confinement. In words prescient of announcements of lockdown during the coronavirus pandemic, Saramago has the Government speaking through a loudspeaker to the inmates as follows:

> *The decision to gather together in one place all those infected, and, in adjacent but separate quarters all those who have had any kind of contact with them, was not taken without careful consideration. The Government is fully aware of its responsibilities and hopes that those to whom this message is directed will, as the upright citizens they doubtless are, also assume their responsibilities, bearing in mind that the isolation in which they now find themselves will represent, above any personal considerations, an act of solidarity with the rest of the nation's community.*
>
> (Saramago, 2013, p. 41)

Away from quarantine works, other literature, memoir or reportage extends land-based confinement to topics such as solitary confinement in prisons, as in Terry Waite's autobiography *Taken on Trust* (1993), recounting his experience of over four years held hostage in a prison cell in Beirut or, more recently, the stories captured in *Six by Ten: Stories from Solitary* (2018), edited by Taylor Pendergrass and Mateo Hoke. In Terry Waite's account, we gain a palpable sense of spatial reduction and the kind of pacing behaviour that solitary confinement provokes:

> *When I opened my eyes, I was in an empty cell lined*
> *with white tiles. I sat down on the floor and looked*
> *around. The room was almost seven feet across and*
> *about ten feet long. The height varied between six*
> *feet and six feet nine. I could be certain about that*
> *because I am six feet seven inches tall and in places it*
> *was impossible for me to stand upright. ... Then I did*
> *what generations of prisoners have done before me. I*
> *stood up and, bending my head, I began to walk*
> *round and round and round and round.*
>
> (Waite, 1993, pp. 7–8)

Throughout the four years of his confinement Waite outlines the battle to retain his sanity with a lack of stimulation only partly relieved by books to read:

> *I have lost track of the days. It's probably Tuesday,*
> *but I can't be sure. One day is very much the same as*
> *another. Bread and lebne for breakfast, one quick*
> *visit to the bathroom, and then twenty-three hours*
> *and fifty minutes lying in the corner with nothing but*
> *my thoughts.*
>
> (Waite, 1993, p. 81)

In a salient observation, Waite recognises the burden of thinking about family while isolated. This is something that many people cut off from loved ones during the pandemic will have experienced to one degree of another:

> *I keep wondering what has happened to my family and friends. I hope my children have continued their education. Whenever my mind goes to those close to me, I get upset. Now I understand why so many long-term prisoners cut themselves off completely from their families. The pain can be too hard to bear.*
>
> (Waite, 1993, p. 201)

We gain a strong sense of the physical deterioration and psychological affliction that can result from prolonged isolation:

> *I am sinking low. My body aches from repeated coughing which I am quite unable to control. My lungs are congested, and for hours on end I fight for breath. … Somehow I have to do two things. I must, if I am going to make any psychological progress whatsoever, continue my interior dialogue. At the same time I have to bolster myself to an almost ridiculous degree. If I let my inner confidence collapse, I will die.*
>
> (Waite, 1993, p. 297)

AT SEA

Although the small spaces referred to as cabins occur on land, in the air and in space, many people will relate to their presence at sea, on ships and most palpably on cruise ships during the pandemic. This kind of naval entrapment became highly publicised in the case of the *Diamond Princess*, a cruise ship which in early 2020 fell foul of coronavirus on its way from Singapore to Japan, eventually being forced to dock for quarantine at Yokohama, Tokyo Bay. Among its 3,711 passengers and crew, 712 tested positive for COVID-19, just under one-fifth of those aboard (Moriarty, 2020). Katie Glass's (2020) account of this voyage captures various narratives of passengers and crew subject to the frightening prospect of contagion without anywhere to run. Even though passengers had built in the spatial limitations of cruising, few expected the eventual isolations in their cabins and for those in the cheapest accommodation this presented a windowless prospect compounded by the fear of infection. As a cruise doctor reported, cruise ships are prone for 'wildfire' infection spread as passengers are effectively contained in a 'metal box' (Glass, 2020, p. 15). According to passenger narratives captured by Glass, who described the setting as a 'floating prison' (p. 16), being captive in their cabins brought very real challenges with boredom, lack of exercise, and establishing a comforting routine to pass the time. While some became creative – for example by starting video diaries – being cooped up was difficult for many. One passenger, David Abel is quoted stating how dire this experience can be: 'You've got no idea of the pressure on board a ship when you are confined to a cabin like this' (Glass, 2020, p. 16). Surprisingly perhaps, one passenger, Alan Sandford, found the subsequent experience of social lockdown more challenging than naval quarantine in his cabin:

> *Quarantine on board the ship is different to isolation at home. In quarantine you are under very strict restrictions, but everything is done for you and you are all in it together. Now we are all in it together, but having to cope separately.*

(Glass, 2020, p. 17)

Here, Sandford distinguishes between physical and notional 'togetherness', suggesting that in lockdown the negative effects of social isolation are compounded by a lack of intimacy and human contact. Physical togetherness is surely the kind of buffer to isolation that many sailors across history welcomed on long voyages.

Experiencing long journeys on steamships in days gone by in small, possibly lightless cabins below deck on transatlantic crossings, in long-distance solo sailing, beneath the sea in submarines, or possibly more luxurious accommodation on the latest cruise ships, whether at sea or held in quarantine in or outside ports, conjures up the potential mental duress of confinement and claustrophobia. In the following wood engraving, for example, we see apprehensive passengers on a ship undergoing quarantine examination during the Egyptian cholera epidemic of 1883 (Fig. 3.2).

We begin to imagine long drawn out periods of unwanted time, unrelenting bland seascapes or oppressive notions of people trapped or imprisoned. As an extreme and tragic case, one can only begin to imagine the torment of the 23 crew of the ill-fated Russian submarine *Kursk* which sank in 2000. The intensity of their confinement after the initial explosions and sinking of the vessel must have been unbearable. Less dramatically perhaps, but nonetheless highly anxiety provoking, those caught up on cruise ships during the pandemic faced significant physical and psychological challenge. Quite aside from the pandemic, advertisements for cruises give the game away about the risk of boredom onboard with their foregrounding of the many activities on offer. The pandemic has certainly proven to be a stress test of the notion of cruising for fun. Indeed, both passengers and sailors working on cruise ships worldwide faced big hits during the pandemic with sickness and deaths from the virus and further tragic conse-quences as some seafarers succumbed to deteriorating mental

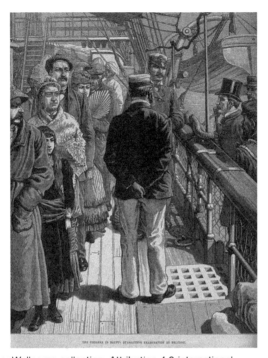

Source: Wellcome collection. Attribution 4.0 international.

Fig. 3.2. Passengers on a Ship Undergoing Quarantine Examination during the Egyptian Cholera Epidemic of 1883. Wood Engraving, 1883.

health and took their own lives. The following image of the *World Dream* arriving into quarantine at Kai Tak Cruise Terminal looks the very opposite to fun (Fig. 3.3).

Writing on the dilemma faced by cruise ships denied entry to port, such as the *Zaandam*, *Diamond Princess* and *Grand Princess*, Roorda (2020) comments: 'COVID-19 would hijack a cruise ship like a legion of invisible pirates' spreading easily through the densely populated environment from 'roomy penthouses to kennel-like crew quarters'. Bywater (2020) reports that the cruise ship *Stella Australis*, blocked from

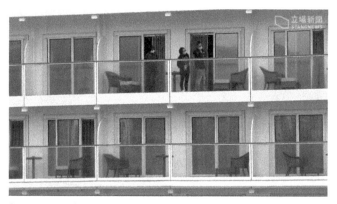

Fig. 3.3. Cruise Ship Quarantine: World Dream Arrives at Kai Tak Cruise Terminal.

entering port in Chile despite no one onboard having coronavirus, succumbed to widespread cases of cabin fever caused by prolonged boredom. Mustoe and Profitt (2020) reported on the dire situation for an estimated 150,000 seafarers from different countries stuck on oil tankers, container ships and cruise ships long after passengers got off at various ports. Without a clear indication of how long quarantine would apply to them and being held at sea indefinitely without shore leave proved too much of a burden. One officer reports:

> *Morale is quite low, especially because you can't go out ashore and without that by definition it's cabin fever … You're working all the time in the same environment, everyone's groggy, everyone wants to go home, people start making small mistakes and it gets you down. We are trying our best to get along with each other.*

(Mustoe & Profitt, 2020, n.p.)

Unfortunately, reports followed of hunger strikes and even suicides of stranded crew. There were cases of crew jumping to their death overboard, for example, a 39-year old woman on the *Regal Princess*, held off the Netherlands, and a crew member from the *Jewel of the Seas* (Greenfield & McCormick, 2020; Street, 2020). This particular behaviour marks a blurring between the kind of desperate psychological state that can result from cabin fever and delirious states associated with actual bodily fever contracted at sea, in the tropics, as described until the nineteenth century as 'calenture'.

There has been much written on contracting infection at sea, not least typhus, that provides a parallel development in cabin fever-related symptoms and behaviour as that which we outlined in regard to land. The Merriam-Webster dictionary points to the affliction of calenture, dating back in first usage to 1582. Here the resulting delirium from this condition affecting sailors is described in striking terms:

> *In addition to being plagued by scurvy and homesickness, sailors of yore who dared the tropics also had calenture to worry about. Given a case of this fever they were likely to imagine that the sea was actually a green field and to leap into it. Our earliest evidence of the word in English is from the late 16th century. Such potent imagery destined the word for figurative use also. 'Calenture' has its origins in a Spanish word of the same meaning, 'calentura,' which itself traces to Latin* calēre, *meaning 'to be warm.' Other words from 'calēre' include 'calorie,' 'cauldron,' and 'scald.'*

> (Merriam-Webster, n.d.)

As we noted earlier, delirium and stupor feature as symptoms in both actual physical fever or pyrexia and the psychological 'fever' or restlessness induced in cabin fever. The delirium induced hallucination of the sea as a green field to be jumped into became literally a colourful trope rather than a medically supported symptom. As Macleod (1983) indicated, this behavioural phenomenon and deluded impulse to leap into the sea has a curious history, dropping out of psychiatric literature in the nineteenth century. He pinpoints the early use of the term *Paraphyrosyne Calentura* by Francois Bossier de Sauvages (1771) for this frenzied action and also cites Falret (1839) who, he writes, 'considered calenture to be a psychological consequence of environmental factors peculiar to sailors – the weather and sea conditions, and the over-crowded living quarters' (Macleod, 1983, p. 347). Various writers such as Jonathan Swift, Daniel Defoe, John Donne, Erasmus Darwin, Samuel Johnson and Herman Melville referred to, defined, or used it as a dramatic trope (see Bewell, 1999; Cheshire, 2018; Mabee, 2017). Wordsworth exploited it in his pastoral 'The Brothers', in the figure of Leonard Ewbanks who experiences the condition. As Frank Mabee articulates: '[He] draws on the literary history of calenture as a signifier for the tropics and for the less salubrious aspects of the colonial trade' (Mabee, 2017, p. 136).

Calenture, or 'the calenture' as some commentators put it, is what William Ingalls refers to as 'ship fever' (Ingalls, 1848, p. 21), linking it to typhus contracted by sailors in the tropics but also more generally to outbreaks on crowded ships. As we may expect in the early period of scientific understanding when medicine debated miasmas ahead of advances in microbiology, Ingalls, like Lyons a little later in 1878, high-lights the quagmire of definition surrounding the term fever, never mind 'ship fever': 'Men of comprehensive minds, of deep research, and profound erudition, have failed to give a comprehensive and perfectly satisfactory definition of fever' (Ingalls, 1848, p. 5). The diversity in fever lends itself to caution in separating out historical and literary reference to an affliction that crossed physical and psychological domains. This is palpable in early theorising on fever that focussed on it as a condition affecting the brain and nervous system as much as other bodily parts as then understood and perhaps goes some way to explain the conjoined evolution of terms such as 'cabin fever' and 'calenture' marking both disturbed physical and psychological equanimity.

Macleod (1983) does not outlaw the possibility of people feeling compelled or lured to jump into the sea despite the weak psychiatric evidence, not least from knowledge of the deleterious impact of sensory deprivation on mental health that may occur on becalmed seas, as in the Doldrums, with 'a horizon devoid of life' (p. 348) and reports of subjective experiences of fusion with extreme, devoid environments among high altitude pilots, polar explorers and mountaineers. This presents as a 'breaking off' detachment or lost connection with one's more immediate and familiar reality (see Clark & Graybiel, 1957). He also flags up a survey by the National Union of Seamen (1981), identifying 15% (577) of the 3,778 deaths occurring at sea between 1964 and 1978 as attributable to homicide (61), suicide (279) and 'missing at sea' (237) (MacLeod, 1983, p. 348).

Yet in the absence of substantive, contemporary research accounting for the folk syndrome 'cabin fever' or even what is termed 'calenture' or 'ship fever' from a nautical perspective, we now turn to a few narratives of experiencing confinement or isolation at sea and representation of how this impacts on mental health or even, sadly, provokes the tragedy of suicide. Narratives about such feverish or frenzied responses will help us to fill in the gaps. What is compelling is that, regardless of the science, people respond badly to confinement at sea as much as land.

The first person to sail solo, non-stop, around the world in 312 days, faced the challenge of extended isolation in a limited space and the risk to his mental health. In an interview report by Robertson and Ramsay (2018) for CNN, commemorating 50 years since his epic voyage, Knox-Johnson advises that you have to be 'stubborn' to do this and that he kept his mind active and sane by learning poetry:

> *I missed the human contact, not being able to discuss things with someone. I just had to sit there and have the conversation with myself—it's actually quite hard to argue with yourself.*

In his travel memoir of the journey, *A World of My Own*, (1969), reissued in 2020, Knox-Johnson writes of the challenge:

> *I wondered if I could manage that long without human company, or if I would go round the bend.*
>
> (Knox-Johnson, 2020, p. 2)

Later, only a month into the voyage that would cause him to hallucinate human voices, he points up the challenge of isolation on his mood and efforts to assuage boredom. As with Terry Waite, books partly mitigated the experience:

> *Some of the problems associated with loneliness and having to do absolutely everything for oneself were beginning to appear. Normally, when I have a number of jobs that need to be done, I take the one that most suits my mood at the time. This would not do now; I had to do things at once or when the weather was favourable regardless of my mood. Then, too, if there was nothing urgent to be done, and no job that could occupy my time, I found myself*

> *getting bored and books would only act as a*
> *temporary stopgap. I would get restless and long for*
> *the voyage to be over, and it was not until October*
> *that I found I had come to accept at all*
> *philosophically that I was to spend perhaps a year of*
> *my life in this way.*

(Knox-Johnson, 2020, p. 51)

Similarly, another sailor, Kevin Farebrother, taking on the 2018 Golden Globe Race, admits loneliness as the core test:

> *This is a huge challenge and probably the hardest*
> *thing I've ever done. It's the whole endurance thing,*
> *it's the whole package about whether I can deal with*
> *the loneliness, whether I can deal with what's ahead*
> *in the Southern Ocean.*

(Robertson & Ramsay, 2018)

Of course, not all sailors sail alone. Sailing crew can suffer cooped up onboard. The claustrophobic nature of life at sea, stuck in cabins and subject to the close company of others, is powerfully conveyed in William Golding's *Rites of Passage* (1980), which becomes the first part of *To the Ends of the Earth: A Sea Trilogy* (1991). Seen through the eyes of the first-person narrator Edmund Talbot, we witness a growing unease and encroaching madness among many of those on board. Talbot diagnoses the dangers of life at such close quarters:

> *With lack of sleep and too much understanding I*
> *grow a little crazy, I think, like all men at sea who*
> *live too close to each other and too close thereby to*
> *all that is monstrous under the sun and moon.*

(Golding, 1980, p. 278)

As the voyage progresses in Golding's novels *Close Quarters* (1987) and *Fire Down Below* (1989) which complete his 'sea trilogy', behaviour deteriorates, and the vessel becomes a Ship of Fools, a restricted space of incarcerated, confined and unhinged people subjected in the Doldrums to their own encircling, stinking effluence. With the death by shame of the clergyman Colley for sexual impropriety to Wheeler's suicide in Colley's cabin, Golding examines the impact of naval entrapment on the human mind.

Jennifer Niven's *The Ice Master* (2001) provides a powerful account of this intense experience of entrapment onboard the *Karluk* in her reportage of Viljalmur Stefansson's ill-fated Canadian Arctic Expedition in 1913, drawing on letters and journals. The wooden ship ended up, terrifyingly, trapped in an ice sheet and only 14 of the original crew of 25 people survived. The crew faced claustrophobia amid a looming, unending icescape. The threat of inactivity and stasis started to impact on the seafarers (Fig. 3.4):

> *By late August it was clear that the men of the* Karluk *were trapped. The seventeen-degree-Fahrenheit temperature seemed even more bitterly cold. The imprisoned ship was drowning in snow. The wind blasted them from all directions, forever shifting and changing course. Inside the* Karluk, *they were warm, but the air was close and stale. The world around them was vast and wide–open sky, ice as far as the eye could see in all directions, nothing to obstruct their view of that boundless, frozen wonderland. But they began to feel claustrophobic. They felt smothered by ice, as if it were not only compressing the sides of their ship, but constricting their throats, and the breath in their lungs.*
>
> *'How long will this continue?' wrote McKinlay. 'This … inactivity is becoming unbearable. The ice even*

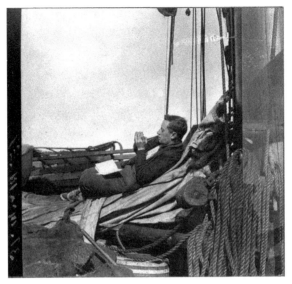

Credit: Library and Archives Canada/Rudolph Martin Anderson and Mae Bell Allstrandfonds/PA-203460.

Fig. 3.4. William L. McKinlay aboard *Karluk*.

reflects the general state of affairs; there is not the slightest sign of movement in it. The small patches of open water have frozen up & all is as still & quiet as death. In the minds of all is the unuttered question, 'When will things change?' Will the change come soon?

(Niven, 2001, p. 45)

The trapped crew are comforted by their sanctuary while opposingly terrified that the ship might be crushed under the pressure of the surrounding ice. Restlessness and conflict grow in the confined space. They endeavour to pass the time and stay busy but they struggle to counter 'a dreary, aimless existence' (Niven, 2001, p. 49), with violent arguments breaking out. The compounding loss of light, something that intensifies cabin fever in remote northern winters, Ernest Chafe, the assistant steward wrote:

> *So long as the sun was with us to measure the night and day, it was not so bad but when the orb disappeared, a sort of sickening sensation of loneliness came over us.*

> (Niven, 2001, p. 5)

To buffer cabin fever the crew engaged creatively, singing, dancing and even putting on a sports program on the ice. Eventually, when the ship was finally lost to the ice they then had to take their chances finding land on their sleds.

IN THE AIR

Some air passengers are known to suffer with panic or unruly behaviour which has been described in lay terms of 'cabin fever', 'air rage' or 'sky rage' (see Bor, 1999; Dahlberg, 2016; Hunter, 2009; Reuters, 2015; Thomas, 2001). As Vredenburgh, Zackowitz, and Vredenburgh (2015) note, aggressive passengers during flights are a real problem causing diverts and unscheduled landings. Quite aside from the obvious impact of alcohol on aggression, the authors identify various key irritants relating to lack of space that provokes rage, not least unroomy or confined seating which forces unwanted proximity with others. Such proximity inevitably brings raised tension around the use of armrests due to passenger obesity or other factors resulting from being at 'close quarters', such as unwanted seat reclining, unpleasant smells and children kicking the back of seats. Also, passengers have to contend with limited access to restroom space, poor storage in overhead bins leading to conflict over possessions and other stressors such as flight delays, meagre food and intrusive noise. In their survey they found that over one-third of the participants were 'more agitated when flying than in their typical life' (p. 403) and concluded: 'Space is a significant problem that needs to be addressed. It is the key issue that has caused reported conflict in this study' (p. 404). Alison Tonks (2008) examines in-flight emergencies and identifies that these are stressful not least because of the restricted environment: 'There's not much light, it's hard to lie someone flat, the seats are cramped, and it's noisy'. In this cooped up or claustrophobic environment and feeling aggrieved in some way, we can begin to see a resemblance between air rage, road rage and cabin fever.

In the air at least, part of feeling aggrieved may be put down to class divide as DeCelles and Norton (2016) suggest. They argue that the 'modern airplane is a social microcosm of class-based society, and that the increasing incidence of "air rage" can be understood through the lens of inequality' (p. 5588). They conclude: 'As both inequality and class-based airplane seating continue to rise, incidents of air rage may similarly climb in frequency' (p. 5590). Effectively, they find that air rage is more common in economy class on flights that have first-class seating, indicating that the status of being a 'have not' exacerbates irritability (Fig. 3.5). We may surmise, on this basis, that the contrast of first-class space versus economy space primes for conflict. Whether we focus on the class division or not as exacerbatory, as Dahlberg (2016) notes:

> [For] the cabin class passenger, the increasingly restricted space between rows can lead to a feeling of personal space being invaded, and for the already claustrophobic individual, that further magnifies the stress.
>
> (p. x)

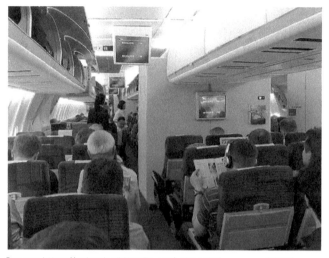

Source: https://upload.wikimedia.org/wikipedia/commons/0/06/
Finnair_MD-11_Economy_class_cabin.jpg.

**Fig. 3.5. Finnair MD-11 Economy Class Cabin. Waldec from
Tallinn, Estonia. Derivative Work: Altair78.**

This powder keg of an environment may become even
more tense in the context of the pandemic with passengers
nervous about people sneezing, coughing, making contact
with their bodies or failing to protect others by wearing face
masks.

There may be other factors at play with cabin fever experiences in the air. As we noted earlier, high altitude pilots may
join other isolated individuals at sea, in wild landscapes or on
mountains in the 'break-off phenomenon' (Clark & Graybiel,
1957) in which they experience fusion with their environments
and detachment from their immediate reality. As Clark and
Graybiel indicate, such pilots can perceive themselves as 'very
much alone and somehow losing their connection with the
world' (p. 122). How far we can or should ascribe such

detachment to aviation's version of cabin fever is yet to be ascertained. Do passengers experience a 'breaking off' to the point in being lured to open plane doors (even if they cannot do so due to internal air pressure mid-flight) as dramatically as sailors seeking to jump into the ocean, mountaineers from mountains or polar explorers racing off into the whiteness? Just one of many such incidents involved a woman feeling claustrophobic opening the cabin door for relief from the stuffy air as the plane stood on the tarmac at Wuhan Tianhe International Airport, China (Murdock, 2019). More dramatically, perhaps, Coffey (2020) reports on a man who had to be forcibly restrained when attempting to open a plane door mid-flight. This compulsion to escape the cabin may place the individual or a group in jeopardy even though air pressure countermands the danger.

Notably, Clark and Graybiel report that the feeling of isolation or loneliness accompanied 71% of those high altitude pilots in their study who had experienced 'breaking off'. The loneliness of piloting more generally, and not just at high altitude, features in the writing of Sir Francis Chichester who completed long-distance solitary journeys by air and sea. Earlier in 1929 he conducted a solo flight in his de Havilland Gipsy Moth from England to Australia. He wrote of the isolation both in the air and at sea in his travel memoir, *The Lonely Sea and Sky* (1964), quite likely referencing the Douglas test pilot William Bridgeman's *The Lonely Sky* (1956). Chichester's desire for company is clear when he chooses the pronoun 'we' when flying solo and capturing the depressing loneliness of these combined environments:

> *We flew through the curtain of rain into an immense cavern of space between the illimitable vault of dull sky above, and the immeasurable floor of dull water below. It was solitary in that great space. Some*

> *slanting pillars of rain leaned against the wind,*
> *trailing across the dull floor of water like spirits of*
> *the dead drifting from the infernal regions. The*
> *vastness lent it all a nightmare air.*
>
> (Chichester, 2002, p. 203)

Among literary representations of the experience of confinement in the air, the thriller genre offers tension in stories of flights subject to hijacking by terrorists on the ground or in mid-air or air rage. John J. Nance's offering in *Turbulence* (2002), for example, tells the story of increasingly irritated passengers driven to air rage and mutiny. We can also read a more light-hearted flight attendant account of the phenomenon in Elliot Hester's *Plane Insanity* (2003). Other genres such as memoir or reportage provide stories of surviving extreme elements alone or in competition with others in the miserable confines of an airwreck. An example of the latter is Piers Paul Read's harrowing account, *Alive: The Story of the Andes Survivors* (1974), which tells the story of a plane lost in the remote Andes mountains carrying a team of rugby players with 25 family and friends. The mental duress of isolation and conflict experienced by the surviving 16 passengers huddled together for three months in the 'confined cabin' (Read, 2012, p. 11) of the broken fuselage, and stark, barely thinkable, actions to stave off hunger by eating their dead (anthropophagy) is extreme. They became even more cooped up following an avalanche. The loss of space is palpable:

> *As night set in, the survivors were wet, cramped, and*
> *bitterly cold, with no cushions, shoes or blankets to*
> *protect them. There was barely room to sit or stand;*
> *they could only lie in a tangle, punching each other's*
> *bodies to keep the blood flowing in their veins, yet*

> *not knowing to whom the arms and legs belonged.*
> *To make more space, some of the snow in the centre*
> *of the cabin was shovelled to either end.*

(p.148)

Unsurprisingly, perhaps, living in such confined quarters brought conflict, with individuals alienated from or infuriating others.

IN SPACE

Astronauts have endured long periods of time in space, as much as six months at a time, for example, on the International Space Station (ISS). Astronauts have had to learn how to get along with other members of the crew in a highly restricted cabin. Retired Canadian astronaut Chris Hadfield offered his advice for people dealing with coronavirus isolation based on his experience of occupying confined spacecraft surrounded by endless and dangerous space. Hadfield maintains that in the current pandemic 'everybody's getting a little taste right now just how isolated it would be to be part of that crew that lands on Mars' (Hadfield, 2020).

Pagel and Choukèr (2016) examined the impacts in diverse long-duration space flight in terrestrial analogue studies, finding human psychology and physiology are 'significantly altered by isolation and confinement' (p. 1449). They foreground the signal case of how during the winter of 1956 a team member at the US Amundsen-Scott Station at the South Pole developed paranoid schizophrenia, ending up being sedated until such a time as he could be transferred out. This provoked psychiatric screening for missions to Antarctica. In their review they conclude: 'Isolation and confinement can put

the human body under a large amount of psycho-
neuroendocrine duress, which results in measurable patho-
physiologic symptoms' (p. 1455). According to the authors,
participants 'subjected to these space analog conditions can
encounter typical symptoms ranging from neurocognitive
changes, fatigue, misaligned circadian rhythm, sleep disorders,
altered stress hormone levels, and immune modulatory
changes' (p. 1449).

Similarly, an assessment of the feasibility of a human
mission to Mars in 2033 commissioned by NASA found
human isolation to be a major challenge independently but
also synergistically with other stressors (Linck et al., 2019).
The report noted the limited evidence of impacts of missions
longer than six months. The report states that so far only six
US astronauts had accumulated more than one year equiva-
lent in space but none exceeded a single mission of more than
one year. Since an extended Mars mission is estimated to last
some 1,100 days (Connolly, 2017), the report clearly indicates
we do not yet know what the impact might be on health. Of
the health risks, the report considers cognitive and behavioural aspects as a high risk category. Citing the Hawaii Space
Exploration Analog and Simulation isolation experiments
from the University of Hawaii, isolation experienced on ISS,
research in Antarctica and the Mars 500 mission, the report
concludes that while we know more about the real challenges
in group dynamics for sustained periods of isolation, and as
yet no astronaut to date has died for health-related reasons,
there remains concern that the much longer duration in space
required to get to Mars might bring new and unforeseen
physical and psychological jeopardy. The extended time spent
in space by astronauts to date suggests that the challenge can
be met. For example, the Russian astronauts Gennady
Padalka achieved a world record for spending the longest time
in space at 879 days over five missions, while Valeri Polyakov

secured the longest single stay at 437 days and 18 hours on board Mir Space Station. Similarly, the US astronaut Peggy Whitsen accumulated 665 days in space (Keating, 2017). Even so, with the much longer duration that a trip to Mars will entail, the threat of cabin fever remains severe. A stark and sobering reminder of the risk is clear in the case of an Argentinian doctor who burned down the Almirante Brown Antarctic base to escape another winter in isolation (Walker, 2013).

The Mars Desert Research Station (MDRS) based in the Utah desert has been investigating the impact of isolation on humans. MDRS simulates a Mars environment as much as this is possible on earth and researchers psychologically investigate the way humans respond to the inhabited space and isolation (Fig. 3.6). Popovaite (2020a, 2020b) identified

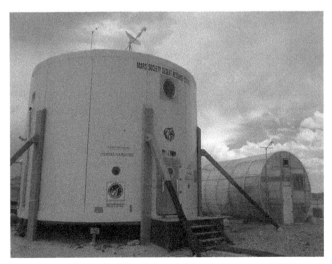

Source: https://upload.wikimedia.org/wikipedia/commons/3/36/
Mars_Desert_Research_Station.jpg.

Fig. 3.6. Mars Desert Research Station (McKay Salisbury).

gender and crew domination issues in such environments and considered the coronavirus isolation as instructive concerning isolation on future space missions. In particular, she identifies differences in stressors, relationships and sexual behaviour. Worryingly, her study found that social and gender inequalities and cultural stereotypes perseverate in mixed crew isolation, including, for example, sexual harassment of women and male domination of important tasks such as simulated space walks. The domination of women in this context corroborates contemporary findings on increased domestic violence during the coronavirus outbreak as noted in the opening chapter.

Lawrence A. Palinkas, who conducted a number of studies into psychosocial aspects of space flight, concluded that stress due to isolation and confinement impacted significantly on cognition and emotion: 'For many individuals, the prospects of living and working in an isolated, confining and hostile environment for prolonged periods of time can be quite stressful' (Palinkas, 2001, p. 25). Salient challenges include many aspects that mirror the social isolation during the pandemic such as separation from loved ones, limits on communication, lack of privacy and personal space, social monotony or boredom, territoriality and interpersonal conflict or hostility. Palinkas usefully summarises reports in prior literature from space flight missions, space simulators and polar research stations as revealing an increase in symptoms of irritability/anger, depression, anxiety, insomnia, fatigue and reduced cognitive performance in prolonged isolation, not least in over-wintering. In an earlier study, Palinkas, Gunderson, Johnson, and Holland (2000) identified both possibilities of conflict or cohesion in groups living in prolonged social isolation with normative microcultures appearing to develop best in smaller, less diverse groups, subject to flexible leadership rather than domination.

In Daniel Oberhaus's (2015) compelling review of the possibilities for sex in space he notes the dangers it poses for social dynamics in confinement:

> *Understanding how sex impacts small-group dynamics in isolation is a crucial component to its successful integration as a variable into missions to space. When small crews are forced to spend months or years in close confinement, figuring out ways to tolerate one another's presence and cooperate can prove to be very taxing. Having two love birds along for a ride might only complicate things further.*
>
> (n.p.)

He writes that such isolation can provoke sexual activity as noted in pregnancies that Australian researchers documented at Antarctic research stations. While married couples appear to stabilise interpersonal relationships in confined groups (Leon, 2005; Leon & Sandal, 2003), this may not always be the case.

The full extent of the impact of confinement on sexual relationships with married couples or singles and how this relates to conflict in space or otherwise remains underexplored. Sheridan Prasso (2020) reports on the 'divorce spike' in China after quarantine in the coronavirus outbreak. For one interviewee, the 'marital irritants' included 'money (too little), screen time (too much), and housework and child care (not evenly split)'. Prasso reports increased domestic violence during lockdown, writing: 'If absence makes the heart grow fonder, the opposite might be true of too much time spent together in close quarters'. The correlation between quarantine or lockdown and domestic violence has been observed in several countries since the outbreak (Faiola & Herrero, 2020). However, Prasso rightly notes that, conversely, many couples have been growing closer during isolation. Clearly, much more research on the social dynamics of marital and sexual relationships in confinement is required when considering long-duration space missions as that proposed in the trip to Mars (Koerth, 2017).

Various works of science fiction represent experiences of being trapped or isolated in spaceships or on distant planets. For example, Andy Weir's novel, *The Martian* (2011), which served as the basis for the 2015 film starring Matt Damon, tells the story of astronaut Mark Watney's extreme isolation and resilience after being stranded in a temporary base, named *Hab*, on the red planet. The crew aborted the mission in their spacecraft *Hermes*. This cabin fever appetizer that exploits current NASA plans to send people to Mars and one of many fictions that focus on the tension of being confined, isolated, or lost in space.

> So that's the situation. I'm stranded on Mars. I have no way to communicate with Hermes or Earth. Everyone thinks I'm dead. I'm in a Hab designed to last thirty-one days.
>
> If the oxygenator breaks down, I'll suffocate. If the water reclaimer breaks down, I'll die of thirst. If the Hab breaches, I'll just kind of explode. If none of those things happen, I'll eventually run out of food and stave to death.
>
> So yeah. I'm fucked.
>
> (Weir, 2011, p. 7)

Watney's plight is relieved through his ingenuity, eventually linking up communications with Earth but not before a period of intense, palpable abandonment, having spent 'three months as the loneliest man in history' (p. 115).

We can experience such extreme isolation themes in other sci-fi literature. Arthur C. Clarke's short story, *Thirty Seconds – Thirty Days* (1949), which also became a film *Trapped in Space* (1994), tells the claustrophobic, tragic tale of how damage to a space freighter and resulting oxygen depletion led to tormented efforts at survival. After Captain Grant's failed attempt to poison McNeil to get the chance to return safely alone with the last of the oxygen, he agrees to commit suicide and McNeil is rescued after enduring three weeks isolated on the stricken vessel. Clarke's novel and script (with Stanley Kubrick) *2001: A Space Odyssey* (1968), extended the kind of claustrophobic tension that we find in cabin fever as HAL takes over, proceeding to exterminate the crew. Peter Hamilton's *The Abyss Beyond Dreams* (2014) tells the tale of humans and aliens trapped in the Void, a structure at the centre of the Milky Way galaxy. While Stephen Baxter's novel *Titan* (1997) explores extreme isolation of an in-fighting crew of astronauts slowly dying out on Saturn's moon, Titan.

A different kind of sci-fi work powerfully salient to the current pandemic lockdown is Isaac Asimov's short story *It's Such a Beautiful Day* (1955). Set in a futuristic San Francisco where teleportation negates the need for physically leaving homes, schoolboy Dickie Hanshaw wanders outside and gets a cold. His mother seeks psychiatric assessment, from Dr Sloane, perceiving her son's behaviour as abnormal. Despite his concerns, Dr Sloane joins the boy in walking outdoors and learns to appreciate this now dispreferred activity.

Whether trapped, abandoned or isolated in space, all these stories evoke various kinds of confinement and turns of intense loneliness. What we find as a theme in fiction also appears in behind-the-scenes reportage such as Chris Jones's *Out of Orbit* (2008). In this account, previously published as *Too Far From Home*, we learn the plight of two American astronauts, Donald Pettit and Kenneth Bowersox, and Russian flight engineer Nikolai Budarin, left orbiting Earth in the ISS and initially unable to return home after the Columbia shuttle fell apart.

Jones identifies that the isolation for the crew of three astronauts on Expedition 66 waiting for their ticket home was not entirely oppressive and by all accounts they found 'the best parts of lonely', appreciating the freedom from more relationally complicated life down on earth and passing the time as productively and positively as possible. Instead of moping, Jones writes:

> *They spent their time busily turning their desert island into more of a paradise than a prison. Together, they rededicated themselves to making [the] station into a sanctuary, and to figuring out how they might stay hidden away for a long time in it.*

(p. 163)

With no ride home, they knew they had to counter the very real psychological and physical challenges ahead. As Jones observes, the threat of mental decline in space is very real:

> *Although the American space program has traditionally paid little attention to the psychological health of its astronauts in space–and most astronauts have been reluctant to discuss any problems they might have had in orbit, lest it harm their prospects for future assignments–there is strong evidence that spending a long time in space can make people crackers. Weeks and months of interrupted sleep, sensory deprivation, isolation, confinement, latent danger, poor hygiene, lousy food, chronic noise and vibration, and close permanent contact with fellow crew members ... Not surprisingly, that wretched mix has proved fertile ground for a host of disorders to take root.*

(p. 175)

He continues:

> *While the vast majority of astronauts and*
> *cosmonauts repel complete psychological*
> *breakdown, many have suffered from fatigue,*
> *nervousness, weakness, anger, and memory and*
> *motor hiccups. In addition to the innate power of*
> *space to push emotions toward the margins of*
> *acceptability, it also tends to bring out the worst in*
> *its inhabitants. More often than not, space will*
> *expose cracks that are invisible on the ground. It can*
> *see through masks and bravado.*

(p. 175)

Despite the best efforts of the astronauts to create a sanctuary, the nagging isolation was such that when they had a film night, complete with popcorn, the film's overstimulation brought intense anxiety.

> *Bowersox, Petit, and Budarin looked down at their*
> *hands, and they were shaking. Their mouths had*
> *gone dry. Their hearts galloped. Every biological*
> *stress indicator had kicked into overdrive. None of*
> *them made it to the end of the movie for fear of*
> *system failure. Together, they agreed to turn it off, to*
> *talk to one another in whispers, and to take a little*
> *longer than usual to come down before going to bed.*
> *But even after they'd tried to unwind and pulled*
> *themselves into their sleeping bags, they still*
> *trembled, like wide-eyed kids who've been told ghost*
> *stories around a campfire before lights-out.*

(p. 179)

It appears that the astronauts had started to go down with cabin fever. As Jones writes:

> *Come morning, they had each drawn the same*
> *conclusion: despite their gut wishes, maybe they had*
> *been gone for long enough. Maybe they needed to*
> *start thinking about going home. Maybe they needed*
> *to answer the questions of when and where and how.*
> *Maybe it was time.*
>
> *Because the earth had been spinning on its axis, and*
> *they had been spinning on theirs, but now they knew*
> *that they'd been travelling in opposite directions for*
> *all of this time, and they felt as though they had never*
> *been so far away.*

(p. 179)

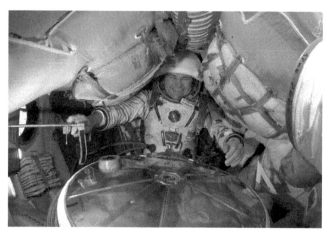

Source: https://upload.wikimedia.org/wikipedia/commons/3/3d/ISS-06_Nikolai_Budarin_in_the_Soyuz_TMA-1_spacecraft.jpg; NASA.

Fig. 3.7. Nikolai Budarin in the Soyuz TMA-1 Spacecraft [Kenneth D. Bowersox Bottom Right].

It would remain a highly stressful time as they had to put their hope in an outdated and very suspect *Soyuz TMA-1* capsule for their escape from the ISS, moving from one small uncertain confinement to another, even more hazardous and tiny 'padded-box'. In the following image we see the bravado of Nikolai Budarin in the claustrophobic capsule with Kenneth D. Bowersox. Bowersox looks decidedly less bullish (lower right). What is particularly striking about the image is just how cramped the space looks without the third member of the crew even being in shot (Fig. 3.7).

4

ANTIDOTES TO CABIN FEVER

Dealing with and managing such a folk syndrome as cabin fever tends, as Rosenblatt, Anderson, and Johnson (1984) note, to be through self-help or support groups rather than any direct medical, psychiatric or psychological intervention. Yet, as we saw earlier, symptoms that feature in cabin fever do attract medical and psychological attention, not least in studies of how individuals and groups adapt to restricted spaces or routines for long periods in, for example, prisons, remote settings, on ships, planes or even spacecraft. Indeed, there has been considerable effort to understand how confinement, not least in restricted spatial environments, impacts on human health and well-being. The pandemic led to a renewed interest and concern about the physical and psychological dangers of lockdown. In turn, many commentators began to offer their best advice for mitigating the effect of confinement and isolation. In this chapter, we consider the kinds of antidotes to the folk or culture-bound syndrome of cabin fever. In light of the pandemic, the term antidote seems apposite, not least given the way that cabin fever has been relatable to both physical infection and psychological duress.

The notion of antidotes to any kind of fever or contagion is not new of course. Across the history of plague, pestilence and multiple other afflictions, people have been offered all kinds of elixirs, remedies or cures. Most of these have been spurious and generated by widespread quackery. Quacks, or charlatan doctors, have always muddied the waters as to what is good for human health and how best to treat ailments. The origin for the term quackery appears to derive 'from the Dutch "quicksalver", meaning a quicksilver doctor, since mercury was widely used to treat syphilis' (Porter, 1999, p. 284). In desperate times especially, people have spent their money on all kinds of ineffectual and even dangerous potions or treatments. As Roy Porter (1999, 2001) notes, a great variety of nostrums were advertised and made available, with only some of these genuinely contributing to managing symptoms. In the enlightenment of the eighteenth century, ironically, the availability of fake medicine and other healing interventions increased with consumer demand. In what Porter calls this Golden Age of quackery, charlatans purveyed their goods on the street in eye-catching, dramatic shows, drawing on tales of exotic origins for their product. In an etching by J. Franklin we see people strolling and buying 'infallible' remedies in old St Paul's Cathedral, London (Fig. 4.1). Fake medicine, then, or being taken in by quacks, has had a lively history long before achieving the relative stability of evidenced-based healthcare in the contemporary period. It is to contemporary evidence of what mitigates cabin fever that we focus on in this chapter.

Writing about isolation in space, retired astronaut Scott Kelly (2020) suggests a number of helpful responses to the challenges of living for long periods in quarantine on earth. First, having a schedule or plan provides a structure that assists adjustment to living alone or with family members. Second, pacing activities, ensuring a balance between work and leisure. Third, keeping to a consistent bedtime, best protecting healthy

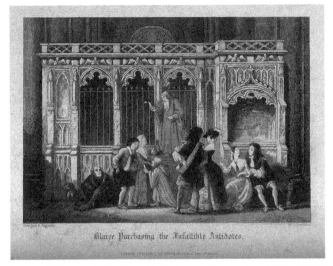

Blaize Purchasing the Infallible Antidotes.

Fig. 4.1. People Strolling and Buying Plague Antidotes in Old St Paul's Cathedral, London. Etching by J. Franklin.

cognition, mood and relationships. Fourth, getting outside in nature and exercising. Fifth, having an outlet or hobby, for example, reading, playing an instrument or arts and crafts to afford 'much-needed unplugged time'. Sixth, keeping a journal to capture experiences, memories and reflections during this exceptional, historical period. Seventh, making use of the technology to connect with family and friends. Eighth, trusting the advice of experts and 'reputable sources of facts' to keep you and your family safe and well. Finally, exploring compassionate behaviour to extend beyond our own personal needs to those of neighbours.

In similar fashion, Bottolier-Depois (2020) collates tips for 'staving off cabin fever' during lockdown from both astro-nauts and submariners. Key among these are having a regular schedule to counter 'suspended time', avoiding the temptation to look too far ahead (counting the days), sharing a mission to 'navigate this ordeal', exercise, accessing nature where possible, trying new creative things, rejecting guilt when facing drop-offs in morale and productivity, and maintaining communication with others, even if this is only electronically. The more obvious treatment or therapy for cabin fever to mitigate or buffer against negative impacts of prolonged isolation or lack of stimulation is to reverse or ameliorate the stressors of confinement. This may be achieved through non-confinement in the open air or less restrictive spaces or the introduction of novel or stimulating activities. In this chapter, we discuss these and other protective behaviours. We examine what can be called green or nature-based remedies, the physical and psychological adjustments that people can make and the value of creative practices in the arts and humanities for survival during lockdown.

GREEN OR NATURE-BASED REMEDIES

As much as nature can challenge us, for example in severe weather or pandemics, we have a deep affinity to it (Wilson, 1984). We recognise that it can heal as well as hurt us. Increasingly, urban populations seek the 'great outdoors', conversing with nature in sometimes idiosyncratic ways and bringing nature into their homes and onto their balconies. People value parks and other green spaces as recreational assets visited and revisited time and again. Beautiful landscapes and seascapes drive the global holiday industry and our passion to indulge in nature. When access to nature and its green or multicoloured vistas is impeded or removed, even temporarily, humans can feel uncomfortable. At worst, subject to long periods of confinement, discomfort can turn into distress. In cabin fever, the indoors–outdoors tension is intense, and the obvious solution quickly springs to mind.

A change of scenery may be as simple as providing access to the outdoors, be it a prison exercise yard, a garden or wider urban or rural scenery, and, importantly, nature. Nature, with its green spaces and sunlight, can be restorative and buffer our mental health, bolstering our immune function, reducing the stress hormone cortisol and lowering blood pressure (see, for example, Alcock, White, Wheeler, Fleming, & Depledge, 2014; Communities and Local Government Committee, 2017; Gascon et al., 2015; Genuis, 2006; Hägerhäll et al., 2015; Jennings, Larson, & Yun, 2016; Kaplan & Kaplan, 1989; Larson, Jennings, & Cloutier, 2016; Ulrich, 1981; Ulrich et al., 1991). Even hearing the sounds of nature can enhance well-being (Alvarsson, Wiens, & Nilsson, 2010; Nilsson & Berglund, 2006; Ratcliffe, Gatersleben, & Sowden, 2013).

During the pandemic, there were many reports on the changes in noise levels from reduced traffic flow and how bird song and other sounds of nature became more audible (Fears, 2020; Keena, 2020; Koren, 2020). Birds moved more freely across roads, darting in and out of residential hedgerows. People with gardens took the opportunity to spend more time in them, either occupying themselves by cutting the lawn, sorting the borders and suchlike or passively enjoying being out in nature. Others have turned to birdwatching or taking more interest in trees and plants, or indeed the sky unmarked by vapour trails. Birds, flowers and sky became symbols of freedom just as they are in penal environments.

While nature and access outdoors is the logical and first line antidote in cabin fever, when the external environment is dangerous, for example in space, during harsh weather, or as in the case for this book, a pandemic, we need to find ways to endure being indoors. This can prove highly challenging. It requires physical and psychological adjustments to a spatially restricted environment. Although nature is typically viewed as an outdoor as opposed to an indoor phenomenon, this is not necessarily the case. The benefits of nature can be brought indoors through enjoyment of internally placed flora and fauna, and virtual nature through image, video or sound. The latter opens a window on perhaps more creative aspects to surviving social isolation or responding to cabin fever.

ACCEPTING THE NEW NORMAL

A key psychological response to enforced isolation indoors is acceptance. Each individual or group needs to self-talk or share a frame or determination to normalise the unusual situation. In other words, we need to find ways to accept the 'new normal'. To accept and adapt to the new normal, of course, may require changing behaviour or taking new protective steps. For example, for people who are ordinarily anxious, subject to depression or other compounding psychological states, this may require reducing exposure to news feeds on the pandemic and avoiding keywords on social media which may trigger being afraid and feeling overwhelmed or hopeless; staying connected with family or friends with regular 'check-in' arrangements; and balancing routine and variety through the day (Brewer, 2020). In addition, there is a wealth of therapeutic literature available online or by referral for managing anxiety, depression or dealing with other mental health conditions, such as Obsessive Compulsive Disorder (OCD) which may be challenging at a time when hand washing is recommended and fears of contamination abound or eating disorders when the media places great emphasis on weight gain during lockdown.

SOCIAL CONNECTEDNESS

We noted earlier in the book the profound impact that social isolation can have on mental health in non-pandemic or pandemic contexts. We established that social connectedness is important in maintaining good mental health. Clearly, social contact has been disrupted in lockdown with people adjusting how they can meet family members, friends or the wider public at this time. The loss of social connectedness during lockdown will be different for individuals under social distancing restrictions depending on where and how these are applied. People from different countries, regions of countries and urban or rural localities will experience varying parameters for maintaining or developing their social interaction. Some will have entered lockdown alone, while others will have company. Many individuals will have contracted the virus with various consequences for communicating with others. For those with access to technological resources such as mobile phones or computers, the challenge of restricted face-to-face, physical meetings with family and friends may have been significantly mitigated. For those without the succour of social media due to their personal circumstances, lockdown could present a major challenge. Yet, tragically, some people will find themselves with company or social connectedness that is damaging, as witnessed in domestic violence and abuse. That said, we can say in general terms that being able to connect and engage with others is an important antidote to cabin fever. Anything that can be done to achieve a level of social interaction that meets individual needs will be worth pursuing.

GOAL SETTING AND PURPOSE

It is important to set achievable goals to motivate and reward activity over lassitude (the loss of physical and mental energy) when faced with prolonged confinement and reduced social connectedness. Although passive activities, such as watching movies or television shows, can be cathartic and help to relieve stress (Schlozman, 2020), these activities need to be balanced with more structured, purposeful approaches. Remaining productive, mentally occupied and physically active can mitigate enforced confinement. A change in physical or mental activity and routine is important and has proven health benefits. This can be achieved through introducing new resources for individual or group occupation and interest. It can be as simple as having a different kind of drink or meal or revisiting an activity that used to bring pleasure. Striking a balance between a daily routine and surprising ourselves with new activities brings purpose and variety.

This focus on purpose is powerfully conveyed in Zweig's (1941) novel, *Chess*, discussed earlier. Dr B responds creatively to the unremitting dullness of his extreme social isolation in a hotel by dividing up his day and filling time by playing chess in his mind after stealing a book of championship matches from one of his interrogators. However, even this, without variation, eventually compromises Dr B's mental state. In a kind of monomania, he ends up paradoxically, impossibly playing chess against himself, losing connection with reality, failing to eat and drink. The importance of variety and balance as a buffer to social isolation is the message we might take from this fiction.

Retired Canadian astronaut Chris Hadfield (2020), in another instalment of advice for households on how to cope with lockdown, stressed the need to act like a crew with purpose each day. He goes on to suggest planning for the day ahead by breaking it up into chunks of activities that need to get done, which will give individuals a sense of pride and accomplishment.

SANCTUARY VERSUS PRISON

For many people, especially those with serious underlying health conditions, their homes during lockdown may begin to feel more of a sanctuary than a prison. In turn, they may struggle at the end of a lockdown period to return to the outside world. They may have become used to the security of their environment despite its spatial or social limitations and prefer to retain this over perceived risk of infection should they step outside again. This may even be the case when infection rates are low enough to allow for more social activities. For others, such as Jennifer Toon, a former prison inmate, the non-penal lockdown can bring a feeling of unwelcome and unfair additional incarceration. She reflects poignantly on how during lockdown she began to feel she was back in prison or under 'house arrest' again. In those penal incarcerations, she had battled not to lose her mind 'from being entombed and cut off from the world' (Toon, 2020, n.p.). Importantly, she identifies her adjustment to such confinement as a shift in mentality that offered the development of a new, deeper inner world. This positive view of solitude changed her perspective, converting the prison cell into a refuge and sanctuary. During lockdown, she suggests, it is better if people can see the restriction not as simply being locked in but locking out disease.

It was this kind of effort that we noted earlier with the astronauts Bowersox, Petit and Budarin, trying to preserve a positive mentality about their confinement on the International Space Station. While this might not completely counter the psychological challenges of prolonged lockdown, especially for those with underlying health conditions who had to shield themselves for longer than the general population, it would appear to be a robust strategy for mitigating its impacts.

For some people, achieving a sanctuary includes spiritual expression or worship which itself has been compromised during lockdown. Places of worship such as churches, mosques, temples and synagogues have remained closed or under strict rules limiting physical public attendance. However, the pandemic has clearly brought a wealth of new digital opportunities for experiencing both spiritual and secular shared meaning making in the face of the pandemic, its threats and resultant isolation. In terms of the former, for example, multiple online opportunities emerged for people to witness and share their faith. In terms of the latter, we can perhaps see social media extending a bubble of sanctuary much wider in a safe way. While there have been frequent warnings about people being 'always on' and electronically connected with others (e.g. Baron, 2008), the pandemic has underlined this communicative resource during lockdown. Frankly, one wonders how much worse lockdown would have been without diverse virtual outreach, kisses and hugs. We may also wonder what kind of 'altered behavioural and social norms' (Baron, 2008, p. 4) around our use of communicative technology will result from the pandemic and experience of lockdown.

LOOKING AFTER THE BODY

It is very well established that exercise, good nutrition (including hydration) and sufficient sleep underpin general health, and this is all the more important during the pandemic to ensure our bodies are better placed to meet the immuno-logical and physical hit the virus places on us. This is especially the case with those who are overweight, have reduced immune function due to increased age or other serious underlying health conditions such as poor cardio-respiratory function, high blood pressure or diabetes. Such individuals face a much higher risk of needing intensive care support if infected. Exercise and good nutrition are also pillars of psychological health. If we are physically inactive or under-nourished and dehydrated, our mental health can also be compromised.

We know that exercise releases endorphins or happy chemicals and improves our chances to fight off infection or deal with compromised functionality. Of course, in small dwellings without access to gardens or when exercise outdoors beyond the garden is not possible we need to make adjustments and innovate to remain active. Exercise within closed spaces features in survival in prolonged imprisonment in cells and prison yards. Following gym closures in the pandemic, people joined online workouts, adapted to home-based exercise or exercised locally or further afield under different phases of the lockdown. At one point, a UK Government health advice advert showed a film of a man running up and down domestic stairs to maintain the standard notion of 10,000 step exercise efficacy. Ironically, this did not foreground the risk of falling down stairs, a common accident leading to hospital admission; something most people wanted to avoid during the pandemic! A more iconic and celebrated modelling of the value of exercise, of course, came with the example of Captain Sir Tom Moore, a centenarian knighted for raising over £30m for National Health Service charities by taking up his family's challenge to walk with the aid of his zimmer frame the length of his garden 100 times to celebrate his birthday.

Maintaining healthy eating and hydration is also important in the face of the virus. While hydration may be easily sorted in those households with potable tap water, access to healthy, nutritious food and the range of vitamins and minerals required for optimal immune function and our core bodily functions has not always been easy, particularly for low-income individuals and families. While many people may have been able to maintain good levels of exercise and a balanced diet of healthy food and drink during the pandemic, others have struggled to protect their physical and psychological health in this way. In terms of nutrition, this has been exacerbated during the pandemic with food banks and other hunger relief organisations globally having to deal with increased demand and operational and public health challenges (Butler, 2020; George & Houreld, 2020; Knott, 2020; Kulish, 2020; Van der Voort, 2020; Young, 2020).

As we noted earlier, sleep can become severely disrupted during periods of lockdown due to raised anxiety levels and other stressors that the pandemic has brought, not least financial concerns and bereavement. It is well established that poor sleep can compromise both our physical and mental health. Conversely, decent sleep can bring enhanced mood and improved cognitive and immune function. It can buffer against conditions such as high blood pressure, heart disease and diabetes, all of which are significant underlying conditions that make people vulnerable to the coronavirus. In other words, sleep is a great antidote to the virus and the psychological onslaught, cabin fever. Alongside exercise and good nutrition, getting outside when possible is important during lockdown to experience the natural light and dark that underpins the circadian rhythm that makes us sleepy and take to our beds. Daylight also tops up melatonin which regulates our sleep and waking pattern. There are many other things we can avoid to maximise success with the pillow. First, we can reduce the level of stimulation before bedtime by limiting coffee, tea and other caffeinated drinks to the morning only and by avoiding or limiting alcohol intake. These drinks and recreational drugs, including smoking, reduce or interrupt good sleep. Recreational drugs can also compound anxiety states. Second, we should limit the use of laptops, tablets, TVs and smart phones in the run up to bed as blue light tricks the body into thinking it is still daytime and disturbs our internal body clock. Third, we can stop watching anxiety-provoking media such as the news, with its continual trauma stories. Fourth, we can pursue a steady, familiar routine and winding down for our sleep (for example, through dimming lights, listening to soothing music, bathing or reading). To set a routine, it is important to avoid napping and lie-ins to best maintain the circadian rhythm. Various organisations offer these and other additional tips on the best approaches to a good night's sleep (See, for example, NHS, 2020).

So far, we have mostly focused on antidotes that seem more predictable or immediately obvious, perhaps, such as access to nature, setting goals and finding purpose, maintaining social connectedness, exercise, good nutrition, quality sleep and perceiving and developing the sense of home as a sanctuary rather than a prison. We turn now to the notion of creative survival, that is, how engagement in the arts and humanities can act as a key antidote in the fight against cabin fever.

CREATIVE SURVIVAL

In the early weeks of the pandemic lockdown, people from across the world engaged on social media at an unprecedented level, sharing emotions, warnings, solutions and creative resources or assets (Fischer, 2020; Gilsenan, 2020). Vast amounts of stories, film, animation, music, theatre, art and photography emerged from households. This creative wave did not simply move through social media but also in streets, villages, towns, cities and nations around the globe. One example of trying to instil hope was the appearance of colourful rainbows with positive messages in their windows. In Italy, these appeared with the message '*andrà tutto bene*' (Everything will be alright) or in France and other French-speaking territories such as Quebec as '*Ça va bien aller*' (It's going to be okay) (Mignacca, 2020). Various other phrases accompanied these images elsewhere such as 'Be happy', 'Smile' and 'Storms don't last forever' (Paul, 2020) (Fig. 4.2).

In many countries, we witnessed singing by groups or individuals from house and apartment windows, balconies, roofs or online to the wider community. In the United Kingdom, each Thursday across the nation, people stood at the thresholds of their homes and clapped in support of health and social carers. Yet this became more than clapping with people using sticks and bells in a simple, rhythmic, orchestral performance. It became a joyful yet sober *charivari*, not to mock but to celebrate the generosity and sacrifice of others. What occurred, in effect, was 'an outbreak of creativity' which acted as a 'vaccine to boredom' (Crawford, 2020).

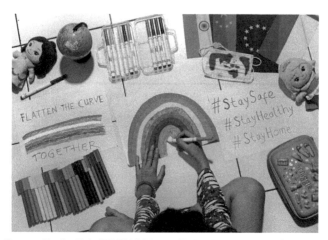

Source: BastianKyle/CC BY-SA https://upload.wikimedia.org/wikipedia/commons/3/39/Stay_Home_for_Our_Safe_and_Healthy_Amid_Covid19.jpg. (https://creativecommons.org/licenses/by-sa/4.0).

Fig. 4.2. Rainbow Art.

During the pandemic, various initiatives looked to support the public's use of creative resources to buffer against mental health problems, notably The MARCH Network's (2020) Creative Isolation initiative and mental health charity Sane's Creative Awards Scheme to fund people with mental health problems to take up a creative activity. As Crawford, Brown, & Charise (2020a) and a new Arts for Health Series (e.g. Davis & Magee, 2020; Irons & Hancox, 2020; Schlozman, 2020) establish, activities such as singing, reading, watching films, dancing and so on can profoundly benefit our physical and mental health. The value of these and other creative activities is also borne out in the accounts of people enduring prolonged confinement, some of which we have captured in this short volume. We also witnessed during the pandemic the development of new applications of creativity such as the design of colourful masks and even personalised scrubs for healthcare staff. Diverse video diaries appeared, and literary agents gathered a slush pile of lockdown novels. In an interview conducted by Philippa Roxby (2020) for BBC news, Kate King, 57, who suffers from anxiety and depression revealed how she responded creatively to social isolation, stating that she 'learnt new ways to cope, centring on living for the day – and playing her melodeon (a squeeze box)'.

At this time of the greatest confinement in history, then, we appear to be witnessing creative practices in the arts and humanities as survival. In thinking through the social and cultural parameters of the new and catastrophic pandemic, there is so much to learn that may inform the future of our societies, how we interact with and comfort each other, and how we cope with mass enforced isolation on an individual and community level. Importantly, we can learn just how vital engagement in the creative arts and humanities can be while the science pursues medical solutions such as effective vaccines. In a creative response to the confinement of cruise ship staff once passengers disembarked, Australian actor Drew Fairley on the *Pacific Explorer*, began a chat show aptly called *Actual Cabin Actual Fever* on Instagram from his cabin on the forlorn ship. He explains:

> *The word cabin fever was being bandied around with everyone staying at home and I was in an actual cabin. So I did a little chat to camera with terrible lighting, just me but in different shirts.*

(Low, 2020, n.p.)

Of course, a change in physical or mental activity and routine can be achieved through more modest and less dramatic approaches. There is a surfeit of low cost physical or online resources for individual or group occupation and interest. Many resources for creativity are already on our person, in our homes, gathering dust in garages or attics, or easily purchased online. Drawing, for example, requires paper, a pencil, a sharpener of some kind and eraser. Singing, dancing and dramatic performance merely requires our bodies, music and imagination. Many crafts can be started with a very modest selection of tools or materials. The current evidence shows that creative practices in the arts and humanities can contribute to survival in social isolation. In an early study on cabin fever Rosenblatt et al. (1984) found 'doing craftwork' helped to break isolation and restrictive routines (p. 50). We know that the creative arts and humanities, including crafts, are powerful contributors to the health of any nation (Crawford, Brown, Baker, Tischler, & Abrams, 2015; Crawford et al., 2020a).

The creative arts and humanities offer a pathway to building resilient individuals and communities, enhancing social connectedness or 'mutual recovery' (Crawford, Lewis, Brown, & Manning, 2013), expression of emotions and thinking, supporting or enhancing our mental health and well-being, and building positive identities. There is, in other words, a social meaning to creativity, which Gauntlett (2011, p. 13) defines as 'activities of making which are rewarding to oneself and to others'; it generates an engaged and engaging citizenry. The last 10 years has seen a flourish of publications, studies and reports underpinning the value of diverse creative activities for our mental health (e.g., APPG, 2017; Arts Council England, 2013; Arts Council of Wales, 2015; Barnett & Fujiwara, 2013; BOP Consulting, 2017; Brown & Kandirikirira, 2007; Cayton & Hewitt, 2007; Coulton, Clift, Skingley, & Rodriguez, 2015; Crawford et al., 2015, 2020a; Department for Culture, Media and Sport, 2016; Fancourt & Finn, 2019; Fujiwara & MacKerron, 2015; Lee, 2013; Ramsden et al., 2011). As Holmes et al. (2020) note, arts-based approaches offer potential mitigation to the mental health burden of the pandemic to enable, among other contributions, 'positive social resources, resilience and altruism'. In other words, creative activities are psychosocially protective as much as aiding physical well-being. These may range from what we commonly think of as mainstream to arts, crafts and humanities practices, for example, dancing, knitting and creative writing, to what have been described as the 'useful arts' of people inventing, making, fixing or building all kinds of things in sheds, garages, workshops or backyards (Crawford, 2009). They are what we should be thinking of as an antidote to cabin fever.

Creative practice is a core aspect of human life. The number and range of creative activities as social and cultural assets globally is staggering. In 2008 in the United Kingdom alone, there were approximately six million people engaged in core visual and other arts, crafts, literature, music and theatre (Dodd, Graves, & Taws, 2013, p. 89). Among the many different creative arts available to the population, reports have counted, for example, 40,000 choirs (Wright, 2017), 11,000 amateur orchestras, 50,000 amateur arts groups, 5,000 amateur theatre societies and 3,000 dance groups (Dodd et al., 2013). Even nearly 20 years ago, there were 50,000 book clubs in the United Kingdom (Hartley, 2001). This is clearly just the tip of a creative iceberg of activities in the arts, crafts and humanities around the world. In addition, digital creative activities, have increased exponentially during the pandemic. The reach of some of these activities has been global rather than national, regional or local as in Eric Whitacre's 'Virtual Choir' (https://ericwhitacre.com/the-virtual-choir).

What has been clear is that in response to the pandemic, many people, not least those living with mental health conditions, have sought refuge in the creative arts in their broadest, inclusive sense. Just as Holmes et al. (2020) raised the importance of arts-based interventions to mitigate against the social isolation and emotional hit of the pandemic, we see large numbers of the public falling back on and taking comfort in artistic or creative endeavours or making. This was the case for the author (PC) who coped with isolation through active and passive engagement in the arts, crafts and humanities from reading, watching films and listening to music through to dancing (alone with disco lights) to keep fit, creative writing, drawing and painting. For example, in order to symbolically re-populate his 'cabin', he did an oil painting of his three children setting off into an abstracted, ghostly, pandemicised Times Square (Fig. 4.3).

Creative coping or survival, that is, enduring or combatting spatial restrictions or routines through activities in the arts and humanities, will play out rather differently for individuals and groups. Broadly, individuals will choose whether to pursue creative activities alone or with others. Clearly, engaging with others can increase social connectedness which we know is protective of mental health yet people may wish to retain a private envelope for their creativity in the midst of others – an escape from sociality and welcome opportunity for

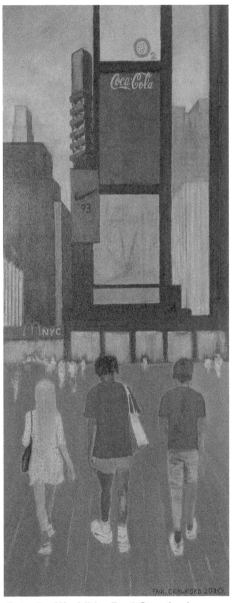

Fig. 4.3. 'Into the World' by Paul Crawford.

personal expression. Either way creativity, whether in arts and crafts or humanities, has been a major feature of what we might think of as pandemic culture. Indeed, the unprecedented global confinement of this pandemic has been met with a similarly unprecedented turn to creative activities as a salve and means of connecting with others. People have found many different creative ways to deal with this remarkable global pandemic, supported for the first time in history by extensive digital technologies. In fact, we witnessed an outburst of creativity as the foremost antidote to another first: global cabin fever.

5

CONCLUSION

The greatest confinement in history due to the coronavirus pandemic continues as we finish this book. Around the world, national, regional and local lockdowns are in full swing, and authorities are kept on their toes to avoid catastrophic public health and economic impact. Just as harrowingly as Daniel Defoe reported on plague in seventeenth-century London, people globally are being shut up in their homes, for better or worse, often for worse until a time when a successful vaccine or therapeutic regime can remove the threat. As the death rate mounts and political tensions intensify, we are all left wondering about the future and what kind of 'new normal' will emerge.

As we wait in not-so-splendid isolation, a mental health pandemic has come in the wake of the stubborn virus. With lockdown dragging on, or applied intermittently, millions of people have been surprised by the very real challenge of cabin fever. What has previously remained backgrounded as a culture-bound, folk term, imagined to afflict only people in remote cabins during harsh winters in various wilderness, has now visited large urban and rural populations. For some the isolation, with or without others, is proving unbearable, not least those who cannot cope with increased anxiety and depression, or those subject to violence and abuse in their own homes. On a positive note, it appears that many people have learned new things about themselves or others during this unprecedented incarceration. While many have struggled desperately in lockdown, others have found social and cultural antidotes to mitigate the impact of isolation. Just as José Mujica, the former Uruguayan president and many others imprisoned for long periods (around 13 years in his case), or under a cloud of threat, as, for example, with Terry Waite, such conditions can bring unexpected and long-standing changes in self-understanding and empathy for others. Indeed, for Mujica, his long years under lock and key brought a profound regard for his fellow citizens and for nature. Noting the paradox that adversity, such as prolonged confinement, can bring positive change or growth, he remarked in the film *El Pepe: A Supreme Life*, 'Sometimes what is good is bad and what's bad is good' (Kusturica, 2018). Yet as people dig deep to counter the multiple kinds of bereavement, loss and pain during the pandemic confinement, we should not underestimate the challenge of the 'brain fever' that comes with isolation. If the highly trained, superfit astronauts of Expedition 6, orbiting the earth without a ride home, can experience it, then so can we. Gaining immunity to cabin fever is not possible, and millions of people will need to work hard to overcome it. By the time this book is published, millions of people will have experienced or will still be experiencing this difficult condition. Their best hope will be to remain creative.

REFERENCES

Alcock, I., White, M. P., Wheeler, B. W., Fleming, L. E., & Depledge, M. H. (2014). Longitudinal effects on mental health of moving to greener and less green urban areas. *Environmental Science & Technology*, 48(2), 1247–1255. doi:10.1021/es403688w

Allen-Ebrahimian, B. (2020, March 7). China's domestic violence epidemic. *Axios*. Retrieved from https://www.axios.com/china-domestic-violence-coronavirus-quarantine-7b00c3ba-35bc-4d16-afdd-b76ecfb28882.html

Allington, D., Beaver, K., Duffy, B., Meyer, C., Moxham-Hall, V., Murkin, G., … Wessely, S. (2020a). *Life under lockdown: Coronavirus in the UK*. The Policy Institute, King's College London. Retrieved from https://www.kcl.ac.uk/policy-institute/assets/coronavirus-in-the-uk.pdf

Allington, D., Beaver, K., Duffy, B., Meyer, C., Moxham-Hall, V., Murkin, G., … Wessely, S. (2020b). *The accepting, the suffering and the resisting: The different reactions to life under lockdown*. The Policy Institute, King's College London. Retrieved from https://www.kcl.ac.uk/policy-institute/assets/coronavirus-in-the-uk.pdf

Alvarsson, J., Wiens, S., & Nilsson, M. (2010). Stress recovery during exposure to nature sound and environmental noise. *International Journal of Environmental Research and Public Health*, 7(3), 1036–1046. doi:10.3390/ijerph7031036

American Psychiatric Association. (2000). *Diagnostic and statistical manual of mental disorders* (4th ed., text rev.). Washington, DC: Author.

American Psychiatric Association. (2013). *Diagnostic and statistical manual of mental disorders* (5th ed.). Washington, DC: Author.

Angelakis, E., Bechah, Y., & Raoult, D. (2016). The history of epidemic typhus. *Microbiology Spectrum*, 4(4). doi:10.1128/microbiolspec.poh-0010-2015

APPG. (2017). *All-party parliamentary group on arts, health and wellbeing inquiry report creative health: The arts for health and wellbeing.* Retrieved from https://www.artshealthandwellbeing.org.uk/appg-inquiry/Publications/Creative_Health_Inquiry_Report_2017.pdf

Arts Council England. (2013). *Great art and culture for everyone.* London: Author. Retrieved from https://www.artscouncil.org.uk/sites/default/files/download-file/Great%20art%20and%20culture%20for%20everyone.pdf

Arts Council of Wales. (2015). *Well-being of future generations (Wales) act consultation on the statutory guidance: Response from the arts council of wales.* London: Author. Retrieved from https://collectorplan.arts.wales/sites/default/files/2019-09/Well-being-of-Future-Generations-consultation-response-Oct-2015.pdf

Asimov, I. (1955). *It's such a beautiful day.* New York: Ballantine Books.

Atcheson, J. D. (1972). Problems of mental health in the Canadian arctic. *Canada's Mental Health*, 20(1), 10–17.

Atwood, M. (2002). *Oryx and crake.* London: Virago.

Bal, M., Crewe, J. V., & Spitzer, L. (Eds.). (1998). *Acts of memory, cultural recall in the present*. Hanover, NH; London: Dartmouth College Press.

Ballard, J. G. (1974). *Concrete Island*. London: Jonathan Cape.

Ballard, J. G. (1975). *High rise*. London: Jonathan Cape.

Barnett, M., & Fujiwara, D. (2013). *Towards plan A: A new political economy for arts and culture*. London: Arts Council England. Retrieved from https://www.thersa.org/globalassets/pdfs/reports/rsa-arts-towards-plan-a.pdf

Baron, N. (2008). *Always on language in an online and mobile world*. New York, NY: Oxford University Press.

Bartlett, C. (2020, June 9). Spate of suspected suicides, deaths among crew on cruise ships. *Safety at Sea*. Retrieved from https://safetyatsea.net/news/2020/spate-of-suicides-and-deaths-among-crew-trapped-on-cruise-ships/

Baxter, G. (2009, October 28). The battle to get rid of Irish typhus. *Irish Medical Times*. Retrieved from https://www.imt.ie/opinion/guest-posts/the-battle-to-get-rid-of-irish-typhus-28-10-2009/

Baxter, S. (1997). *Titan*. New York: Voyager.

Bellatin, M. (1994). *Beauty salon. (K. Hollander, Trans.). Translated into English*. San Francisco: City Lights Publishers, 2009.

Belonsky, A. (2017). *The log cabin: An illustrated history*. New York, NY: Countryman Press.

Belonsky, A. (2018). 'Cabin fever' was coined by a woman in 1918. [Blog post]. Retrieved from https://incaseyoureinterested.com/2018/02/06/cabin-fever-was-coined-by-a-woman-in-1918/

Bergon, H. St J. (2009). Cabin fever. *ISLE: Interdisciplinary Studies in Literature and Environment*, *16*(3), 635. doi: 10.1093/isle/isp056

Beutel, M. E., Klein, E. M., Brähler, E., Reiner, I., Jünger, C., Michal, M., … Tibubos, A. N. (2017). Loneliness in the general population: Prevalence, determinants and relations to mental health. *BMC Psychiatry*, *17*(1), 97. doi:10.1186/s12888-017-1262-x

Bewell, A. (1999). *Romanticism and colonial disease.* Baltimore, MD; London: The Johns Hopkins University Press.

BOP Consulting. (2017). *Reading well books on prescription: Evaluation of year 4 – 2016/17*. London: Author. Retrieved from https://tra-resources.s3.amazonaws.com/uploads/entries/document/2480/171009_TRA_RWBoP_Y4_Evaluation_-_Final.pdf

Bor, R. (1999). Unruly passenger behaviour and in-flight violence: A psychological perspective. *Travel Medicine International*, *17*(1), 5–10.

Bottolier-Depois, A. (2020, March 26). In space, at sea: Tips on isolation from the pros. *The Jakarta Post*. Retrieved from https://www.thejakartapost.com/life/2020/03/26/in-space-at-sea-tips-on-isolation-from-the-pros.html

Bower, B. M. (1918). *Cabin fever: A novel*. Boston, MA: Little, Brown and Company.

Brewer, K. (2020, 16 March). Coronavirus: How to protect your mental health. *BBC News*. Retrieved from https://www.bbc.co.uk/news/health-51873799

Bridgeman, W. (1956). *The lonely sky*. London: Cassell.

Brooks, S. K., Webster, R. K., Smith, L. E., Woodland, L., Wessely, S., Greenberg, N., & Rubin, G. J. (2020).

The psychological impact of quarantine and how to reduce it: Rapid review of the evidence. *The Lancet, 395,* 912–920. doi: 10.1016/S0140-6736(20)30460-8

Brown, W., & Kandirikirira, N. (2007). Recovering mental health in scotland. Report on narrative investigation of mental health recovery. *Scottish Recovery Network*. Retrieved from https://scottishrecovery.net/wp-content/uploads/2008/03/ Recovering_mental_health_in_Scotland_2007.pdf

Brown, B., Rutherford, P., & Crawford, P. (2015). The role of noise in clinical environments with particular reference to mental health care: A narrative review. *International Journal of Nursing Studies, 52*(9), 1514–1524. doi:10.1016/ j.ijnurstu.2015.04.020

Butler, P. (2020, May 1). UK food banks face record demand in coronavirus crisis. *The Guardian*. Retrieved from https:// www.theguardian.com/society/2020/may/01/uk-food-banks-face-record-demand-in-coronavirus-crisis

Bywater, T. (2020, March 26). Coronavirus: Keeping cabin fever at bay on a quarantine ship in Chile. *New Zealand Herald*. Retrieved from https://www.nzherald.co.nz/travel/ news/article.cfm?c_id=7&objectid=12319456

Cambridge Dictionary. (n.d.). Cabin fever. Retrieved from https://www.collinsdictionary.com/dictionary/english/cabin-fever

Campbell, S. J. (1994). *Great Irish famine: Words and images from the Famine Museum, Strokestown Park, County Roscommon*. Strokestown: National Famine Museum.

Camus, A. (1947). *The plague. [La Peste]*. Paris: Gallimard.

Carey, B. (2020, May 19). Is the pandemic sparking suicide? Psychiatrists are confronted with an urgent natural experiment, and the outcome is far from predictable. *New York Times*. Retrieved from https://www.nytimes.com/2020/05/19/health/pandemic-coronavirus-suicide-health.html

Cather, W. (1913). *O pioneers!* Boston, MA: Houghton Mifflin.

Cayton, H., & Hewitt, P. (2007). *A prospectus for arts and health*. London: Arts Council England. Retrieved from http://www.artsandhealth.ie/wp-content/uploads/2011/09/A-prospectus-for-Arts-Health-Arts-Council-England.pdf

Centre for Mental Health. (2010). The economic and social costs of mental health problems in 2009/10. Retrieved from https://www.centreformentalhealth.org.uk/sites/default/files/2018-09/Economic_and_social_costs_2010_0.pdf

Charrière, H. (1969). *Papillon*. Paris: Robert Laffont.

Cheshire, P. (2018). *William Gilbert and esoteric romanticism: A contextual study and annotated edition of 'The Hurricane' (romantic reconfigurations: Studies in literature and culture 1780–1850)*. Liverpool: Liverpool University Press.

Chichester, F. (2002). *The lonely sky and sea*. Chichester: Summersdale. (Original work published 1964).

Christensen, R. (1984). Cabin fever: A folk belief and the misdiagnosis of complaints. *Journal of Mental Health Administration, 11*, 2–3. doi:10.1007/BF02829015

Christopher, J. (1977). *Empty world*. New York: E. P. Dutton.

Clark, B., & Graybiel, A. (1957). The break-off phenomenon. *The Journal of Aviation Medicine, 28*, 121–126.

Clarke, A. C. (1949, December) Thirty seconds – Thirty – Days. In S. Merwin Jr. (Ed.) *Thrilling wonder stories* (pp. 106–122). New York: Standard Magazines.

Clarke, A. C. (1968). *2001: A space Odyssey*. London: Hutchinson.

Clemmer, D. (1940). *The prison community*. New York, NY: Holt, Rinehart and Winston.

Coffey, H. (2020, March 4). Passenger tries to open plane door during flight before being forced to ground and restrained with cable ties. *The Independent*. Retrieved from https://www.independent.co.uk/travel/news-and-advice/passenger-opens-plane-door-flight-american-airlines-restrained-chicago-dallas-st-louis-a9374331.html

Collins English Dictionary. (n.d.). Cabin fever. Retrieved from https://www.collinsdictionary.com/dictionary/english/cabin-fever

Communities and Local Government Committee. (2017). *Public parks, seventh report of session 2016–17*. London: House of Commons. Retrieved from https://publications.parliament.uk/pa/cm201617/cmselect/cmcomloc/45/45.pdf

Connolly, J. (2017). Deep space transport (DST) and Mars mission architecture. *NASA*. October 17. Retrieved from https://nvite.jsc.nasa.gov/presentations/b2/D1_Mars_Connolly.pdf

Constitutional Rights Foundation. (2010). The potato famine and Irish immigration to America. *Bill of Rights in Action*, 26(2). Retrieved from https://www.crf-usa.org/bill-of-rights-in-action/bria-26-2-the-potato-famine-and-irish-immigration-to-america.html

Coon, J. T., Boddy, K., Stein, K., Whear, R. L., Barton, J., & Depledge, M. (2011). Does participating in physical activity in outdoor natural environments have a greater effect on physical and mental wellbeing than physical activity indoors? A systematic review. *Environmental science & technology*, 45(5), 1761–1772.

Coulton, S., Clift, S., Skingley, A., & Rodriguez, J. (2015). Effectiveness and cost-effectiveness of community singing on mental health-related quality of life of older people: Randomised controlled trial. *The British Journal of Psychiatry: The Journal of Mental Science*, 207(3), 250–255. doi:10.1192/bjp.bp.113.129908

Cowan, K. (2020). Survey results: Understanding people's concerns about the mental health impacts of the COVID-19 pandemic. *The Academy of Medical Sciences*. Retrieved from http://www.acmedsci.ac.uk/COVIDmentalhealthsurveys

Coyle, A. (2005). *Understanding prisons*. Maidenhead: Open University Press.

Crawford, M. (2009). *The case for working with your hands: Or why office work is bad for us and fixing things feels good*. London: Penguin Books.

Crawford, P. (2020, May 22). *Coronavirus: An outbreak of creativity*. [Blog post]. Arts and Minds. Retrieved from https://ahrc-blog.com/2020/05/22/coronavirus-an-outbreak-of-creativity/

Crawford, P., Brown, B., Baker, C., Tischler, V., & Abrams, B. (Eds.). (2015). *Health humanities*. London: New York, NY: Palgrave Macmillan. doi:10.1057/9781137282613

Crawford, P., Brown, B., & Charise, A. (Eds.). (2020a). *The Routledge companion to health humanities*. London: Routledge.

Crawford, P., Greenwood, A., Bates, R., & Memel, J. (2020b). *Florence nightingale at home*. London: Palgrave Macmillan. doi:10.1007/978-3-030-46534-6

Crawford, P., Lewis, L., Brown, B., & Manning, N. (2013). Creative practice as mutual recovery in mental health. *Mental Health Review Journal*, *18*(2), 55–64. doi:10.1108/MHRJ-11-2012-0031

Crewe, B., Hulley, S., & Wright, S. (2017). The gendered pains of life imprisonment. *British Journal of Criminology*, *57*(6), 1359–1378. doi:10.1093/bjc/azw088

Crichton, M. (1969). *The Andromeda strain*. New York: Alfred A. Knopf.

Cromartie, J., Nulph, D., Hart, G., & Dobis, E. (2013). Defining frontier areas in the United States. *Journal of Maps*, *9*(2), 149–153. doi:10.1080/17445647.2013.773569

Dahlberg, A. (2016). *Air rage: The underestimated safety risk*. Abingdon: Routledge.

Dancker, J., & Eastwood, J. D. (2020). *Out of my skull: The psychology of boredom*. Cambridge, MA: Harvard University Press.

Davis, P., & Magee, M. (2020). *Reading*. Bingley: Emerald Publishing Limited.

DeCelles, K. A., & Norton, M. I. (2016). Physical and situational inequality on airplanes predicts air rage. *PNAS Proceedings of the National Academy of Sciences of the United States of America*, *113*(20), 5588–5591. doi:10.1073/pnas.1521727113

Defoe, D. (1719). *The life and strange surprizing adventures of Robinson Crusoe* [shortened title]. London: Printed for W. Taylor.

Defoe, D. (1722). *A journal of the Plague year* [shortened title]. London: Printed for E. Nutt. Retrieved from https://www.gutenberg.org/files/376/376-h/376-h.htm

Department for Culture, Media and Sport. (2016). The culture white paper [White paper]. Crown. Retrieved from https://assets.publishing.service.gov.uk/government/uploads/system/uploads/attachment_data/file/510798/DCMS_The_Culture_White_Paper__3_.pdf

Department of Health. (2011). *No health without mental health. A cross-government mental health outcomes strategy for people of all ages*. Crown. London: HM Government. Retrieved from https://assets.publishing.service.gov.uk/government/uploads/system/uploads/attachment_data/file/138253/dh_124058.pdf

Department of Health. (2020). *The mental health impact of COVID-19: An opinion piece by the Australian government's deputy chief medical officer for mental health, Dr Ruth Vine*. Canberra: Commonwealth of Australia, Department of Health. Retrieved from https://www.health.gov.au/news/the-mental-health-impact-of-covid-19

Derby, L. K. (2000). *The great Irish famine: A further understanding of its complexities through the use of human communication theory*. [Doctoral dissertation, Dublin City University]. Retrieved from http://doras.dcu.ie/18496/1/Lisa_Kelly_Derby.pdf

Dick, L. (1995). "Pibloktoq" (Arctic Hysteria): A construction of European-inuit relations? *Arctic Anthropology*, 32(2), 1–42.

Dodd, F., Graves, A., & Taws, K. (2013). *Our creative talent – the voluntary and amateur arts in England*. London: Department for Culture, Media and Sport. Retrieved from https://www.culturehive.co.uk/wp-content/uploads/2013/04/Our-Creative-Talent.pdf

Dosteovsky, F. (1864). Letters from the underworld. *Epoch*, January–April.

Dostoevsky, F. (1866). *Crime and punishment. (D. Magarshack, Trans.). Translated in English*. Penguin: Harmondsworth, 1996.

Duncan, D. (1993). *Miles from nowhere: Tales from America's contemporary frontier*. New York, NY: Penguin.

Durcan, G., O'Shea, N., & Allwood, L. (2020). Covid-19 and the nation's mental health forecasting needs and risks in the UK: May 2020. *Centre for Mental Health*. Retrieved from https://www.centreformentalhealth.org.uk/sites/default/files/2020-05/CentreforMentalHealth_COVID_MH_Forecasting_May20.pdf

Eliot, G. (1863). *Romola*. New York: Harper & Brothers.

Elovainio, M., Hakulinen, C., Pulkki-Råback, L., Virtanen, M., Josefsson, K., Jokela, M., … Kivimäki, M. (2017). Contribution of risk factors to excess mortality in isolated and lonely individuals: An analysis of data from the UK biobank cohort study. *The Lancet Public Health*, 2(6), e260–e266. doi: 10.1016/S2468-2667(17)30075-0

Emmons, D. M. (2010). *Beyond the American pale: The Irish in the west 1845–1910*. Norman, OK: University of Oklahoma Press.

Faiola, A., & Herrero, A. V. (2020, *September 6). For women and children around the world, a double plague: Coronavirus and domestic violence*. The Washington Post. Retrieved from https://www.washingtonpost.com/world/the_americas/coronavirus-domestic-violence/2020/09/06/78c134de-ec7f-11ea-b4bc-3a2098fc73d4_story.html

Falret, J-P. (1839). *Du délire. Dictionnaire des études médicales practiques*. Paris: Société encyclographique des sciences médicales.

Fancourt, D., & Finn, S. (2019). *What is the evidence on the role of the arts in improving health and well-being? A scoping review*. Copenhagen: WHO Regional Office for Europe. Retrieved from https://apps.who.int/iris/bitstream/handle/10665/329834/9789289054553-eng.pdf

Fears, D. (2020, May 22). Amid the pandemic, people are paying more attention to tweets. And not the Twitter kind. *The Washington Post*. Retrieved from https://www.washingtonpost.com/climate-environment/2020/05/22/amid-pandemic-people-are-paying-more-attention-tweets-not-twitter-kind/

Fischer, S. (2020, April 24). Social media use spikes during pandemic. *Axios*. Retrieved from https://www.axios.com/social-media-overuse-spikes-in-coronavirus-pandemic-764b384d-a0ee-4787-bd19-7e7297f6d6ec.html

Foulks, E. F. (1972). *The arctic hysterias of the North Alaskan Eskimo*. Arlington, VA: American Anthropological Association.

Fujiwara, D., & MacKerron, G. (2015). *Cultural activities, artforms and wellbeing*. London: Arts Council England. Retrieved from https://www.artscouncil.org.uk/sites/default/files/download-file/Cultural_activities_artforms_and_wellbeing.pdf

Gallagher, J. A. (1936). The Irish emigration of 1847 and its Canadian consequences. *CCHA Report*, *3*, 43–57. Retrieved from http://www.umanitoba.ca/colleges/st_pauls/ccha/Back%20Issues/CCHA1935-36/Gallagher.html

Garrioch, D. (2003). Sounds of the city: The soundscape of early modern European towns. *Urban History*, *30*(1), 5–25. doi:10.1017/S0963926803001019

Gascon, M., Triguero-Mas, M., Martínez, D., Dadvand, P., Forns, J., Plasència, A., & Nieuwenhuijsen, M. J. (2015). Mental health benefits of long-term exposure to residential green and blue spaces: A systematic review. *International Journal of Environmental Research and Public Health*, *12*(4), 4354–4379. doi:10.3390/ ijerph120404354

Gaskell, E. (1853). *Ruth*. London: Chapman and Hall.

Gauntlett, D. (2011). *Making is connecting: The social meaning of creativity, from DIY and knitting to YouTube and web 2.0*. Cambridge; Malden, MA: Polity Press.

Gayer-Anderson, C., Latham, R., El Zerbi, C., Strang, L., Moxham Hall, V., Knowles, G., … Wilkinson, B. (2020). Impacts of social isolation among disadvantaged and vulnerable groups during public health crises. *ESRC Centre for Society & Mental Health*, King's College London. Retrieved from https://esrc.ukri.org/files/news-events-and-publications/ evidence-briefings/impacts-of-social-isolation-among-dis advantaged-and-vulnerable-groups-during-public-health- crises/

Gelder, M. G., Adreasen, N. C., Lopez-Ibor, J. J., Jr, & Geddes, J. J. (Eds.). (2009). *New oxford textbook of psychiatry* (Vol. 1). Oxford; New York, NY: Oxford University Press.

Gelston, A. L., & Jones, T. C. (1977). Typhus fever: The report of an epidemic in New York city in 1847. *Journal of Infectious Diseases*, *136*(6), 813–821.

Genuis, S. J. (2006). Keeping your sunny side up. How sunlight affects health and well-being. *Canadian Family Physician*, *52*(4), 422–423, 429–431.

George, L., & Houreld, K. (2020, April 16). Millions face hunger as African cities impose coronavirus lockdowns. *Reuters*. Retrieved from https://www.reuters.com/article/us-health-coronavirus-hunger-africa/millions-face-hunger-as-african-cities-impose-coronavirus-lockdowns-idUSKCN21Y14E

Gierveld, J., Tilburg, T., & Dykstra, P. (2018). New ways of theorizing and conducting research in the field of loneliness and social isolation. In A. Vangelisti & D. Perlman (Eds.), *The Cambridge handbook of personal relationships*(Cambridge handbooks in psychology, pp. 391–404). Cambridge: Cambridge University Press. doi:10.1017/9781316417867.031

Gilman, C. P. (1892). *The yellow wallpaper*. New York: Feminist Press.

Gilsenan, K. (2020, July 1). Closely connected: Social media's role during COVID-19. *Global Web Index*. Retrieved from https://blog.globalwebindex.com/trends/social-media-covid-19/

Glass, K. (2020, June 14). Cabin fever. *The Sunday Times Magazine*, pp. 13–17.

Golding, W. (1954). *Lord of the flies*. London: Faber and Faber.

Golding, W. (1980). *Rites of passage*. London: Faber & Faber.

Golding, W. (1987). *Close quarters*. London: Faber & Faber.

Golding, W. (1989). *Fire down below*. London: Faber & Faber.

Golding, W. (1991). *To the ends of the Earth: A sea trilogy*. London: Faber & Faber.

Graham-Harrison, E., Giuffrida, A., Smith, H., & Ford, L. (2020, March 28). Lockdowns around the world bring rise in domestic violence. *The Guardian*. Retrieved from https://www.theguardian.com/society/2020/mar/28/lockdowns-world-rise-domestic-violence

Grantham, P. (2020, April 23). Brits stranded on Panama beach. Interview by A. McVeigh. *BBC News*. London: BBC.

Grebennikov, L., & Wiggins, M. (2006). Psychological effects of classroom noise on early childhood teachers. *The Australian Educational Researcher*, *33*, 35–53. doi:10.1007/BF03216841

Greenfield, P., & McCormick, E. (2020, May 14). Hunger strikes and deaths as mental health crisis grips stranded cruise ships. *The Guardian*. Retrieved from https://www.theguardian.com/environment/2020/may/14/deaths-and-hunger-strikes-point-to-mental-health-crisis-on-stranded-cruise-ships

Gregory, A. (2020, June 21). Coronavirus: Doctors on war footing to tackle surge in PTSD. *The Sunday Times*. Retrieved from https://www.thetimes.co.uk/article/coronavirus-doctors-on-war-footing-to-tackle-surge-in-ptsd-j6hz5sshp

Griffin, J. (2010). *The lonely society?* London: Mental Health Foundation.

Gritsenko, V., Skugarevsky, O., Konstantinov, V., Khamenka, N., Marinova, T., Reznik, A., & Isralowitz, R. (2020). COVID 19 fear, stress, anxiety, and substance use among Russian and Belarusian university students. *International Journal of Mental Health and Addiction*, 1–7. Advance online publication. doi:10.1007/s11469-020-00330-z

Guenther, L. (2013). *Solitary confinement: Social Death and its afterlives*. Minneapolis, MN: University of Minnesota Press.

Gunnell, D., Appleby, L., Arensman, E., Hawton, K., John, A., Kapur, N., … COVID-19 Suicide Prevention Research Collaboration. (2020). Suicide risk and prevention during the COVID-19 pandemic. *The Lancet Psychiatry*, 7(6), 468–471. doi:10.1016/S2215-0366(20)30171-1

Gussow, Z. (1985). Pibloktoq (Hysteria) among the polar eskimo. In R. C. Simons & C. C. Hughes (Eds.), *The culture-bound syndromes* (pp. 271–287). Dordrecht: Springer Netherlands. doi:10.1007/978-94-009-5251-5_26

Gyasi, R. M. (2020). Fighting COVID-19: Fear and internal conflict among older adults in Ghana. *Journal of Gerontological Social Work*. 1–3. doi:10.1080/01634372.2020.1766630

Hadfield, C. (2020, April 3). Chris Hadfield explains how astronauts cope with self-isolation [YouTube]. Retrieved from https://youtu.be/Do-N45kevoE

Hägerhäll, C. M., Laike, T., Küller, M., Marcheschi, E., Boydston, C., & Taylor, R. P. (2015). Human physiological benefits of viewing nature: EEG responses to exact and statistical fractal patterns. *Nonlinear Dynamics, Psychology, and Life Sciences*, 19(1), 1–12.

Hamilton, P. (2014). *The Abyss beyond dreams*. London: Pan Macmillan.

Hardoy, M. C., Carta, M. G., Marci, A. R., Carbone, F., Cadeddu, M., Kovess, V., … Carpiniello, B. (2005). Exposure to aircraft noise and risk of psychiatric disorders: The Elmas survey—aircraft noise and psychiatric disorders. *Social*

Psychiatry and Psychiatric Epidemiology, 40(1), 24–26. doi: 10.1007/s00127-005-0837-x

Hartley, J. (2001). *Reading groups.* Oxford: Oxford University Press.

Hawkley, L., & Cacioppo, J. (2009). Loneliness. In H. T. Reis & S. Sprecher (Eds.), *Encyclopedia of human relationships* (pp. 986–990). Thousand Oaks, CA: SAGE Publishing. doi: 10.4135/9781412958479.n318

Henley, J. (2020, March 28). Lockdown living: How Europeans are avoiding going stir crazy. *The Guardian.* Retrieved from https://www.theguardian.com/world/2020/mar/28/lockdown-living-europe-activities-coronavirus-isolation

Hester, W. (2003). *Plane insanity.* New York: St. Martin's Press.

Holmes, E. A., O'Connor, R. C., Perry, V. H., Tracey, I., Wessely, S., Arseneault, L., ... Bullmore, E. (2020). Multidisciplinary research priorities for the COVID-19 pandemic: A call for action for mental health science. *The Lancet Psychiatry, 7*(6), 547–560. doi:10.1016/S2215-0366(20)30168-1

Holt-Lunstad, J., Smith, T. B., & Layton, J. B. (2010). Social relationships and mortality risk: A meta-analytic review. *PLoS Medicine, 7*(7), e1000316. doi:10.1371/journal.pmed.1000316

Honold, J., Beyer, R., Lakes, T., & van der Meer, E. (2012). Multiple environmental burdens and neighborhood-related health of city residents. *Journal of Environmental Psychology, 32*(4), 305–317. doi:10.1016/j.jenvp.2012.05.002

Hunter, J. A. (2009). *Anger in the air: Combating the air rage phenomenon.* London: Routledge.

IEA. (2020, April). *Global Energy Review 2020: The impacts of the Covid-19 crisis on global energy demand and CO2 emissions*. Retrieved from https://www.iea.org/reports/global-energy-review-2020

Ingalls, W. (1848). *A case of typhus or ship fever, with remarks*. Boston, MA: David Clapp.

Irons, J. Y., & Hancox, G. (2020). *Singing*. Bingley: Emerald Publishing Limited.

Jenness, D. (1928). *The people of the twilight*. New York, NY: Macmillan.

Jennings, V., Larson, L., & Yun, J. (2016). Advancing sustainability through urban green space: Cultural ecosystem services, equity, and social determinants of health. *International Journal of Environmental Research and Public Health*, *13*(2), 196. doi:10.3390/ijerph13020196

Jewkes, Y., Jordan, M., Wright, S., & Bendelow, G. (2019). Designing 'healthy' prisons for women: Incorporating trauma-informed care (TICP) into prison planning and design. *International Journal of Environmental Research and Public Health*, *16*(20), 3818. doi:10.3390/ijerph16203818

Jolley, E. (1991). *Cabin fever: A novel*. New York, NY: HarperCollins.

Jones, C. (2008). *Out of orbit*. New York: Anchor Books.

Jordan, M. (2011). The prison setting as a place of enforced residence, its mental health effects, and the mental healthcare implications. *Health & Place*, *17*(5), 1061–1066. doi: 10.1016/j.healthplace.2011.06.006

Joska, J. A., Andersen, L., Rabie, S., Marais, A., Ndwandwa, E.-S., Wilson, P., … Sikkema, K. J. (2020). COVID-19: Increased risk to the mental health and safety of women living with HIV in South Africa. *AIDS and Behavior, 24,* 2751–2753. doi:10.1007/s10461-020-02897-z

Kanthor, R. (2020, March 18). Under lockdown for coronavirus, parents struggle to deal with their kids. *The New York Times.* Retrieved from https://www.nytimes.com/2020/03/17/parenting/coronavirus-quarantine.html

Kaplan, R., & Kaplan, S. (1989). *The experience of nature: A psychological perspective.* Cambridge; New York, NY: Cambridge University Press.

Karim, F. (2020, April 27). Man in hospital with knife wounds after children, one and three, die in Ilford stabbing. *The Times.* Retrieved from https://www.thetimes.co.uk/article/two-children-one-and-three-killed-in-ilford-stabbing-mjc9hx5ls

Keating, P. (2017, September 3). Astronaut Peggy Whitson breaks NASA's record for longest time spent in space. *The Independent.* Retrieved from https://www.independent.co.uk/news/science/astronaut-peggy-whitsun-nasa-space-international-space-station-world-record-jack-fischer-a7926811.html

Keena, C. (2020, April 17). Coronavirus: Birdsong seems louder and the ravens are more relaxed. *The Irish Times.* Retrieved from https://www.irishtimes.com/news/ireland/irish-news/coronavirus-birdsong-seems-louder-and-the-ravens-are-more-relaxed-1.4231725

Kehoe, J. P., & Abbott, M. B. (1975). Suicide and attempted suicide in the Yukon territory. *The Canadian Journal of Psychiatry, 20*(1), 15–23. doi:10.1177/070674377502000104

Kelly, S. (2020, March 21). I spent a year in space, and I have tips on isolation to share. *The New York Times.* Retrieved from https://www.nytimes.com/2020/03/21/opinion/scott-kelly-coronavirus-isolation.html

Kinderman, P. (2016, March 7). How normal is claustrophobia? *The Independent*. Retrieved from https://www.independent.co.uk/life-style/health-and-families/features/the-truth-about-claustrophobia-a6916596.html

Kinealy, C., & Moran, G. (Eds.). (2019). *The history of the Irish famine: Fallen leaves of humanity: Famines in Ireland before and after the great famine*. London; New York, NY: Routledge.

King, M. R. (1927). The epidemiology of typhus fever in Ireland. *Public Health Reports*, 42(43), 2641. (1896–1970). doi:10.2307/4578547

King, S. (1978). *The stand*. New York: Doubleday.

Kniffen, F., & Glassie, H. (1966). Building in wood in the eastern United States: A time-place perspective. *Geographical Review*, 56(1), 40. doi:10.2307/212734

Knott, K. (2020, May 22). Hong Kong food banks face supply chain disruption, and drop in volunteers and money coming in. *South China Morning Post*. Retrieved from https://www.scmp.com/lifestyle/food-drink/article/3085386/food-banks-supplying-fish-rice-other-essentials-and-meals-hong

Knox-Johnson, R. (2020). *A World of my own: The first ever non-stop solo round the world voyage*. London: Adlard Coles.

Koerth, K. (2017, March 14). Space sex is serious business: We've done almost no research into this area, but it's key to living on Mars. *FiveThirtyEight*. Retrieved from https://fivethirtyeight.com/features/space-sex-is-serious-business/

Koren, M. (2020, April 2). The pandemic is turning the natural world upside down. *The Atlantic*. Retrieved from https://www.theatlantic.com/science/archive/2020/04/coronavirus-pandemic-earth-pollution-noise/609316/

Kulish, N. (2020, May 6). 'Never seen anything like it': Cars line up for miles at food banks. *The New York Times*. Retrieved from https://www.nytimes.com/2020/04/08/business/economy/coronavirus-food-banks.html

Kusturica, E. (2018). *El Pepe: A supreme life*[film]. Kramer & Sigman Films. Oriental Films.

Lancaster-James, H. (2020, April 28). Coronavirus: The psychology of why lockdown is making our relationships stronger. *Sky News*. Retrieved from https://news.sky.com/story/coronavirus-why-the-lockdown-has-made-some-of-our-relationships-stronger-11979709

Landy, D. (1985). Pibloktoq (hysteria) and Inuit nutrition: Possible implication of hypervitaminosis A. *Social science & medicine*, *21*(2), 173–185. (1982). doi:10.1016/0277-9536(85)90087-5

Larson, L. R., Jennings, V., & Cloutier, S. A. (2016). Public parks and wellbeing in urban areas of the United States. *PloS One*, *11*(4), e0153211. doi:10.1371/journal.pone.0153211

Leather, P., Beale, D., & Sullivan, L. (2003). Noise, psychosocial stress and their interaction in the workplace. *Journal of Environmental Psychology*, *23*(2), 213–222. doi: 10.1016/S0272-4944(02)00082-8

Lee, D. (2013). How the arts generate social capital to foster intergroup social cohesion. *The Journal of Arts Management, Law, and Society*, *43*(1), 4–17. doi:10.1080/10632921.2012.761167

Leon, G. R. (2005). Men and women in space. *Aviation Space & Environmental Medicine*, *76*(6), B84–B88.

Leon, G. R., & Sandal, G. M. (2003). Women and couples in isolated extreme environments: Applications for long-duration missions. *Acta Astronautica*, *53*(4–10), 259–267. doi:10.1016/S0094-5765(03)80003-6

Li, D., & Gang, Z. (2020). Psychological interventions for people affected by the COVID-19 epidemic. *The Lancet Psychiatry*, *7*(4), 300–302. doi:10.1016/S2215-0366(20)30073-0

Linck, E., Crane, K. W., Zuckerman, B. L., Corbin, B. A., Myers, R. M., Williams, S. R., … Lal, B. (2019). *Evaluation of a human mission to mars by 2033*. Alexandria, VA: IDA Science & Technology Policy Institute. Retrieved from https://www.ida.org/-/media/feature/publications/e/ev/evaluation-of-a-human-mission-to-mars-by-2033/d-10510.ashx

Li, W., & Schwartzapfel, B. (2020, April 22). *Is domestic violence rising during the coronavirus shutdown? Here's what the data shows*. The Marshall Project. Retrieved from https://www.themarshallproject.org/2020/04/22/is-domestic-violence-rising-during-the-coronavirus-shutdown-here-s-what-the-data-shows

Liu, D., Fernandez, B., Hamilton, A., Lang, N., Gallagher, J., Newby, D., … Weller, R. (2014). UVA irradiation of human skin vasodilates arterial vasculature and lowers blood pressure independently of nitric oxide synthase. *Journal of Investigative Dermatology*, *134*(7), 1839–1846. doi:10.1038/jid.2014.27

Liu, S., Yang, L., Zhang, C., Xiang, Y.-T., Liu, Z., Hu, S., & Zhang, B. (2020). Online mental health services in China during the COVID-19 outbreak. *The Lancet Psychiatry*, *7*(4), e17–e18. doi:10.1016/S2215-0366(20)30077-8

Low, L. A. (2020, April 30). Australian actor stuck at sea turns cabin fever into chat show comedy. *The Sydney Morning Herald*. Retrieved from https://www.smh.com.au/

culture/theatre/stuck-at-sea-this-man-turned-cabin-fever-into-a-one-man-chat-show-20200430-p54oq4.html

Lyons, R. T. (1872). *A treatise on relapsing or famine fever*. London: Henry S. King & Co.

Mabee, F. (2017). The sea as green fields: Calenture and Wordsworth's rural ocean. In S. Mentz & M. E. Rojas (Eds.), *The sea and nineteenth-century Anglophone literary culture* (pp. 135–146). New York, NY: Routledge.

Macleod, A. D. (1983). Calenture—missing at sea? *British Journal of Medical Psychology, 56*(4), 347–350. doi:10.1111/j.2044-8341.1983.tb01566.x

Magarshack, D. (1996). Introduction. (D. Magarshack, Trans.). In F. Dostoevsky (Ed.), *Crime and punishment* (pp. 9–17). New York, NY: Penguin.

Mallen, M. J., Day, S. X., & Green, M. A. (2003). Online versus face-to-face conversation: An examination of relational and discourse variables. *Psychotherapy: Theory, Research, Practice, Training, 40*(1–2), 155–163. doi:10.1037/0033-3204.40.1-2.155

Mandel, St. J. (2014). *Station eleven*. London: Picador.

Márquez, G. G. (1985). *Love in the time of Cholera*. New York: Alfred A. Knopf.

Marsh, S. (2020, July 12). Fifth of vulnerable people considered self-harm in UK lockdown. *The Guardian*. Retrieved from https://www.theguardian.com/society/2020/jul/12/vulnerable-people-self-harm-suicide-uk-lockdown-coronavirus

Martineau, S. (1853). *Sickness and health of the people*. Boston: Crosby, Nichols, and Company.

McDonald, L. (Ed.). (2011). *The collected works of Florence nightingale: Florence nightingale on wars and the war office* (Vol. 15). Waterloo: Wilfrid Laurier University Press.

McGarry, M. (2020). Cabin fever: The dwellings of the rural poor. [Blog post]. Retrieved from https://drmarionmcgarry.weebly.com/irish-heritage-and-identity-blog/cabin-fever-the-dwellings-of-the-rural-poor

Merriam-Webster. (n.d.). Calenture. Retrieved from https://www.merriam-webster.com/dictionary/calenture

Merriam-Webster. (n.d.). Wanderlust. Retrieved from https://www.merriam-webster.com/dictionary/wanderlust

Met Office. (2020, May 29). Spring 2020: The sunniest on record in the UK. [Blog post]. Retrieved from https://blog.metoffice.gov.uk/2020/05/29/spring-2020-the-sunniest-on-record-in-the-uk/

Mignacca, F. G. (2020, April 11). Meet one of the people behind Quebec's 'Ça va bien aller' posters. *CBC News*. Retrieved from https://www.cbc.ca/news/canada/montreal/quebec-ca-va-bien-aller-covid-19-1.5529750

Miles, R., Coutts, C., & Mohamadi, A. (2012). Neighborhood urban form, social environment, and depression. *Journal of Urban Health*, 89(1), 1–18. doi:10.1007/s11524-011-9621-2

Mitchener, J. (1976). *Centennial*. New York: Random House.

Montgomery-Fate, T. (2011). *Cabin fever*. Boston, MA: Beacon Press.

Moriarty, L. F. (2020). Public health responses to COVID-19 outbreaks on cruise ships—worldwide, February–March 2020. *MMWR. Morbidity and Mortality Weekly Report*, 69(12), 347–352. doi:10.15585/mmwr.mm6912e3

Morrison, H. (1987). *Early American architecture: From the first colonial settlements to the first colonial settlements to the national period*. New York, NY: Dover Publications. (Original work published 1905).

Murdock, J. (2019, September 25). Woman detained after opening plane's emergency exit because she needed a 'breath of fresh air' before takeoff. *Newsweek*. Retrieved from https://www.newsweek.com/china-woman-opens-xiamen-air-plane-emergency-door-fresh-air-stuffy-1461286

Mustoe, H., & Proffitt, S. (2020, May 6). Coronavirus: Sailors tell of months stuck on ships. *BBC News*. Retrieved from https://www.bbc.co.uk/news/business-52494839?SThisFB&fbclid=IwAR2R36SoBwLm35HPNnrYdeQeJ4BTMBdP2Jm8HrafohHJ2VrfHW3yUfSig8g

Nance. J. J. (2002). *Turbulence*. New York: Putnam.

NHS. (2020). Ten tips to beat insomnia: Sleep and tiredness. *Crown*. Retrieved from https://www.nhs.uk/live-well/sleep-and-tiredness/10-tips-to-beat-insomnia/

Nilsson, M., & Berglund, B. (2006). Soundscape quality in suburban green areas and city parks. *Acta Acustica United with Acustica*, 92(6), 903–911.

Nitsche, P. H., & Wilmanns, K. (1912). The history of the prison psychoses. *Journal of Nervous and Mental Disease Publishing Company*.

Niven, J. (2001). *The ice master*. London: Pan Books.

Nobles, G. H. (1997). *American frontiers: Cultural encounters and continental conquest*. New York, NY: Hill and Wang.

Norman, K. (1996). Real-world music as composed listening. *Contemporary Music Review*, 15(1), 1–27. doi:10.1080/07494469600640331

Oberhaus, D. (2015, March 30). Let's talk about sex in space. *VICE*. Retrieved from https://www.vice.com/en_us/article/3dky9w/sex-in-space

O'Laughlin, M. (2007). *Missouri Irish: The original history of the Irish in Missouri*. Kansas City: Irish Genealogical Foundation.

Online Etymology Dictionary. (n.d.). Fever. Retrieved from https://www.etymonline.com/word/fever

Orwell, G. (1949). *Nineteen eighty-four: A novel*. London: Secker & Warburg.

Pagel, J. I., & Choukèr, A. (2016). Effects of isolation and confinement on humans-implications for manned space explorations. *Journal of Applied Physiology, 120*(12), 1449–1457. doi:10.1152/japplphysiol.00928.2015

Pagnamenta, P. (2012). *Prairie fever: British aristocrats in the American west*, 1830–1890. New York, NY: W. W. Norton & Company.

Palinkas, L. A. (2001). Psychosocial issues in long-term space flight: Overview. *Gravitational and space biology bulletin: Publication of the American Society for Gravitational and Space Biology, 14*(2), 25–33.

Palinkas, L. A., Gunderson, E. K., Johnson, J. C., & Holland, A. W. (2000). Behavior and performance on long-duration spaceflights: Evidence from analogue environments. *Aviation Space & Environmental Medicine, 71*(9), A29–A36.

Parker, M. F. (2019). *Prairie fever*. New York: Algonquin Books.

Paul, A. (2020, March 25). Coronavirus UK: Why are people putting rainbow pictures on their windows? *Metro News*. Retrieved from https://metro.co.uk/2020/03/25/coronavirus-uk-pictures-rainbows-12454395/

Pendergrass, T., & Hoke, M. (Eds.). (2018). *Stories from solitary*. Chicago: Haymarket Books.

Popovaite, I. (2020a). Coronavirus quarantine could provide lessons for future space travel on how regular people weather isolation. *The Conversation*. Retrieved from https://phys.org/news/2020-04-coronavirus-quarantine-lessons-future-space.html

Popovaite, I. (2020b). Men are from Mars? Gender and crew domination in MDRS simulations. *The Mars Society*. Retrieved from http://mdrs.marssociety.org/research/gender-and-crew-domination-in-mdrs-simulations/

Porter, K. A. (1939). *Pale horse, pale rider*. New York: Harcourt, Brace.

Porter, R. (1999). *The greatest benefit to mankind: A medical history of humanity from antiquity to the present*. London: Fontana Press.

Porter, R. (2001). *Quacks: Fakers and charlatans in English medicine*. Cheltenham: The History Press.

Prasso, S. (2020, March 31). China's divorce spike is a warning to rest of locked-down world. *Bloomberg News*. Retrieved from https://www.bloomberg.com/news/articles/2020-03-31/divorces-spike-in-china-after-coronavirus-quarantines

Putnam, R. D. (2000). *Bowling alone*. New York, NY: Simon & Schuster.

Quehl, J., & Basner, M. (2006). Annoyance from nocturnal aircraft noise exposure: Laboratory and field-specific dose–response curves. *Journal of Environmental Psychology*, 26(2), 127–140. doi:10.1016/j.jenvp.2006.05.006

Ramsden, H., Milling, J., Phillimore, J., McCabe, A., Fyfe, H., & Simpson, R. (2011). *The role of grassroots arts activities in communities*. TSRC Working Paper 68. University of Birmingham, Birmingham, UK. Retrieved from http://epapers.bham.ac.uk/1555/1/WP68_Role_of_grassroots_arts_activities_in_communities_-_McCabe_and_team_Dec_2011.pdf

Raoult, D., Woodward, T., & Dumler, J. S. (2004). The history of epidemic typhus. *Infectious Disease Clinics of North America*, *18*(1), 127–140. doi:10.1016/S0891-5520(03)00093-X

Ratcliffe, E., Gatersleben, B., & Sowden, P. T. (2013). Bird sounds and their contributions to perceived attention restoration and stress recovery. *Journal of Environmental Psychology*, *36*, 221–228. doi:10.1016/j.jenvp.2013.08.004

Read, P. P. (2012). *Alive: There was only one way to survive*. London: Arrow Books. (Original work published 1974).

Reger, M. A., Stanley, I. H., & Joiner, T. E. (2020). Suicide mortality and coronavirus disease 2019—a perfect storm? *JAMA Psychiatry*. doi:10.1001/jamapsychiatry.2020.1060

Renzoni, C. (2020). Common myths about claustrophobia. The Recovery Village Retrieved from https://www.therecoveryvillage.com/mental-health/claustrophobia/related/claustrophobia-myths/

Reuters. (2015). Air rage becoming more common, due to airlines' shrinking seats. *Fortune*. Retrieved from www.fortune.com/2015/04/16/air-rage-becoming-more-common/

Richmond Times-Dispatch. (1918, January 13). *Books and authors. Richmond Times-Dispatch (Richmond, Va.)*, 4. Retrieved from https://chroniclingamerica.loc.gov/lccn/sn83045389/1918-01-13/ed-1/seq-18/

Riesman, D. (1950). *The lonely crowd: A study of the changing American character*. New Haven, CT: Yale University Press.

Robertson, E. (1879). What is the actual condition of Ireland? *Contemporary Review*, *36*(3), 454. Retrieved from http://www.gutenberg.org/files/39517/39517-h/39517-h.htm#Page_454

Robertson, S., & Ramsay, G. (2018, May 11). The first man to sail non-stop solo around the world. *CNN*. Retrieved from https://edition.cnn.com/2018/05/10/sport/golden-globe-race-robin-knox-johnston-round-the-world-sailing-mainsail-spt-intl/index.html

Robinson, M. (1980). Pest house. *Deddington News*, *5*(3). Retrieved from http://www.deddingtonhistory.uk/buildings/pesthouse

Rocha, K., Pérez, K., Rodríguez-Sanz, M., Obiols, J. E., & Borrell, C. (2012). Perception of environmental problems and common mental disorders (CMD). *Social Psychiatry and Psychiatric Epidemiology*, *47*(10), 1675–1684. doi:10.1007/s00127-012-0474-0

Roorda, P. (2020). *Cabin fever: Trapped onboard the last ships at sea*. [Blog post]. Duke University Press. Retrieved from https://dukeupress.wordpress.com/2020/04/03/cabin-fever-trapped-onboard-the-last-ships-at-sea-a-guest-post-by-eric-paul-roorda/

Rorke, P. (1946). *The wisdom of adversity*. London: The Catholic Truth Society.

Rosenblatt, P. C., Anderson, R. M., & Johnson, P. A. (1984). The meaning of "cabin fever". *The Journal of Social Psychology*, *123*(1), 43–53.

Roxby, P. (2020). Coronavirus: 'Profound' mental health impact prompts calls for urgent research. *BBC News*. Retrieved from https://www.bbc.co.uk/news/health-52295894

Sandford, A. (2020, April 2). Coronavirus: Half of humanity now on lockdown as 90 countries call for confinement. *Euronews*. Retrieved from https://www.euronews.com/2020/ 04/02/coronavirus-in-europe-spain-s-death-toll-hits-10-000- after-record-950-new-deaths-in-24-hou

Sansone, R. A., & Sansone, L. A. (2010). Road rage: What's driving it? *Psychiatry (Edgmont (Pa.: Township))*, 7(7), 14–18.

Saramago, J. (2013). *Blindness*. (G. Pontiero., Trans.). London: Vintage Classics.

Schafer, R. M. (1994). *The soundscape: Our sonic Environment and the Tuning of the world*. Rochester, VT: Destiny Books.

Schlozman, S. (2020). *Film*. Bingley: Emerald Publishing Limited.

Schreckenberg, D., Griefahn, B., & Meis, M. (2010). The associations between noise sensitivity, reported physical and mental health, perceived environmental quality, and noise annoyance. *Noise and Health*, 12(46), 7–16. doi:10.4103/ 1463-1741.59995

Serafim, A. de P., Gonçalves, P. D., Rocca, C. C., & Neto, F. L. (2020). The impact of COVID-19 on Brazilian mental health through vicarious traumatization. *Brazilian Journal of Psychiatry*, 42(4), 450. doi:10.1590/1516-4446-2020-0999

Shepherd, D., Welch, D., Dirks, K. N., & Mathews, R. (2010). Exploring the relationship between noise sensitivity, annoyance and health-related quality of life in a sample of adults exposed to environmental noise. *International Journal of Environmental Research and Public Health*, 7(10), 3579–3594. doi:10.3390/ijerph7103580

Sidorov, P. I., & Davydov, A. N. (1992). Ethnopsychiatric research in the national minorities of Northern Russia and Siberia. *The Bekhterev review of psychiatry and medical psychology*.

Sifunda, S., Reddy, P., Braithwaite, R., Stephens, T., Ruiter, R., & van der Borne, B. (2006). Access point analysis on the state of health care services in South African prisoners: A qualitative exploration of correctional health care workers' and inmates' perspective in Kwazulu–Natal and Mpumalanga. *Social Science & Medicine*, 63(9), 2301–2309. doi:10.1016/j.socscimed.2006.06.010

Sims, D. (2020, March 20). 10 perfect films to watch while stuck at home. *The Atlantic*. Retrieved from https://www.theatlantic.com/culture/archive/2020/03/covid19-coronavirus-social-distancing-netflix-hulu/608398/

Slater, P. (1970). *The pursuit of loneliness*. Boston, MA: Beacon Press.

Smith, G. W. (1833). *A defence of the system of solitary confinement of prisoners adopted by the state of Pennsylvania: With remarks on the origin, progress and extension of this species of prison discipline*. Philadelphia, PA: Philadelphia Society for Alleviating the Miseries of Public Prisons.

Sorokin, M. Y., Kasyanov, E. D., Rukavishnikov, G. V., Makarevich, O. V., Neznanov, N. G., Lutova, N. B., & Mazo, G. E. (2020). Structure of anxiety associated with the COVID-19 pandemic in the Russian-speaking sample: Results from on-line survey. *medRxiv*. doi:10.1101/2020.04.28.20074302

Stansfeld, S., & Matheson, M. (2003). Noise pollution: Non-auditory effects on health. *British Medical Bulletin*, *68*, 243–257.

Stowe, H. B. (1852). *Uncle Tom's cabin or life among the lowly*. Boston, MA: John P. Jewett and Company. Retrieved from https://www.gutenberg.org/files/203/203-h/203-h.htm

Street, F. (2020, May 19). Treated as cargo: Stranded cruise ship crews recount desperation. *CNN Business*. Retrieved from https://edition.cnn.com/2020/05/18/health/cruise-ship-mental-health-wellness/index.html

Taub, A. (2020, April 14). A new covid-19 crisis: Domestic abuse rises worldwide. *The New York Times*. Retrieved from https://www.nytimes.com/2020/04/06/world/coronavirus-domestic-violence.html

Teo, A. R., Markwardt, S., & Hinton, L. (2019). Using skype to beat the blues: Longitudinal data from a national representative sample. *American Journal of Geriatric Psychiatry: Official Journal of the American Association for Geriatric Psychiatry*, *27*(3), 254–262. doi:10.1016/j.jagp.2018.10.014

Thakur, V., & Jain, A. (2020). COVID 2019-suicides: A global psychological pandemic. *Brain, Behavior, and Immunity*, *88*, 952–953. doi:10.1016/j.bbi.2020.04.062

The March Network. (2020). Creative isolation. Retrieved from https://www.marchnetwork.org/creative-isolation

Thejesh, G. N. (2020). Non virus deaths. [Blog post]. Retrieved from https://thejeshgn.com/projects/covid19-india/non-virus-deaths/

The Sun. (1918, March 24*). New novels you want to know about. The Sun* (New York, N.Y.), 10. Retrieved from https://chroniclingamerica.loc.gov/lccn/sn83030431/1918-03-24/ed-1/seq-78/'

Thomas, A. R. (2001). *Air rage: Crisis in the skies*. Amherst, MA: Prometheus.

Tonks, A. (2008). Cabin fever. *BMJ* (Clinical research ed.), *336*(7644), 584–586. doi:10.1136/bmj.39511.444618

Toon, J. (2020, April 13). I was in prison for two decades – here's what I learned about isolation. *The Guardian*. Retrieved from https://www.theguardian.com/us-news/2020/apr/13/prison-isolation-coronavirus-pandemic?

Truax, B. (1999a). *Handbook for acoustic ecology* [CD ROM]. Cambridge Street: Records.

Truax, B. (1999b). Composition and diffusion: Space in sound in space. *Organised Sound*, *3*(2), 141. doi:10.1017/S1355771898002076

Truax, B. (2001). *Acoustic communication*. Westport, CT: Ablex.

Truax, B. (2002). Genres and techniques of soundscape composition as developed at Simon Fraser University. *Organised Sound*, *7*(1), 5. doi:10.1017/S1355771802001024

Turkle, S. (2011). *Alone together: Why we expect more from technology and less from each other*. New York, NY: Basic Books.

Turner, F. J. (1893). The significance of the frontier in American history. *Annual Report of the American historical association*. 197–227. Retrieved from https://www.historians.org/about-aha-and-membership/aha-history-and-archives/historical-archives/the-significance-of-the-frontier-in-american-history

Turner, F. J. (1921). *The frontier in American history*. New York, NY: Henry Holt and Company.

Ulrich, R. S. (1981). Natural versus urban scenes: Some psychophysiological effects. *Environment and Behavior*, *13*, 523–556.

Ulrich, R. S., Simons, R. F., Losito, B. D., Fiorito, E., Miles, M. A., & Zelson, M. (1991). Stress recovery during exposure to natural and urban environments. *Journal of Environmental Psychology*, *11*, 201–230.

Underwood, J. O. (1985). Men, women, and madness: Pioneer plains literature. In B. H. Meldrum (Ed.), *Under the sun: Myth and realism in western American literature* (pp. 51–61). Troy, NY: Whitson.

Urban, S. (1820). Review of new publications; letter to the editor of the quarterly review. *The Gentleman's Magazine*, *128*, 137–139.

Van der Voort, Y. (2020, April 23). On the margins of Paris, the food bank queues grow longer. *Reuters*. Retrieved from https://www.reuters.com/article/us-health-coronavirus-france-suburbs/on-the-margins-of-paris-the-food-bank-queues-grow-longer-idUSKCN2251TQ

Varshney, M., Parel, J. T., Raizada, N., & Sarin, S. K. (2020). Initial psychological impact of COVID-19 and its correlates in Indian Community: An online (FEEL-COVID) survey. *PloS One*, *15*(5), e0233874. doi:10.1371/journal.pone.0233874

Vincent, G. (2020, May 6). Charity warns of 'mental illness timebomb' as calls increase by 200%. *ITV News*. Retrieved from https://www.itv.com/news/2020-05-06/charity-warns-of-mental-illness-timebomb-as-calls-increase-by-200/

Visontay, E., & Henriques-Gomes, L. (2020, July 5). 'Explosive potential': Victoria sends 500 police to contain coronavirus in public housing high-rises. *The Guardian*. Retrieved from https://www.theguardian.com/world/2020/jul/

05/explosive-potential-victoria-sends-500-police-to-contain-coronavirus-in-public-housing-high-rises

Vitelli, R. (2020, June 7). Are we facing A post-COVID-19 suicide epidemic? Is the current pandemic putting more people at risk for suicide? *Psychology Today*. Retrieved from https://www.psychologytoday.com/gb/blog/media-spotlight/202006/are-we-facing-post-covid-19-suicide-epidemic

Vredenburgh, A. N., Zackowitz, I. B., & Vredenburgh, A. G. (2015). Air rage: What factors influence airline passenger anger? *Proceedings of the Human Factors and Ergonomics Society - Annual Meeting*, 59(1), 400–404. doi:10.1177/1541931215591084

Waite, T. (1993). *Taken on trust*. London: Hodder and Stoughton.

Walker, T. (2013, August 9). Space: The lonely frontier. *The Independent*. Retrieved from https://www.independent.co.uk/news/world/space-the-lonely-frontier-8754869.html

Wallenius, M. A. (2004). The interaction of noise stress and personal project stress on subjective health. *Journal of Environmental Psychology*, 24(2), 167–177. doi:10.1016/j.jenvp.2003.12.002

Wang, J., Lloyd-Evans, B., Giacco, D., Forsyth, R., Nebo, C., Mann, F., & Johnson, S. (2017). Social isolation in mental health: A conceptual and methodological review. *Social Psychiatry and Psychiatric Epidemiology*, 52(12), 1451–1461. doi:10.1007/s00127-017-1446-1

Warner, K. (2015). *Stir crazy in Kazakhstan*. Bloomington, IN: AuthorHouse.

Weir, A. (2011). *The Martian*. New York: Crown Publishing Group.

Well Being Trust. (2020). Projected deaths of despair from COVID-19. Retrieved from https://wellbeingtrust.org/wp-content/uploads/2020/05/WBT_Deaths-of-Despair_COVID-19-FINAL-FINAL.pdf

Wilson, E. O. (1984). *Biophilia*. Cambridge, MA: Harvard University Press.

Wirz-Justice, A. (2018). Seasonality in affective disorders. *General and Comparative Endocrinology*, *258*, 244–249. doi: 10.1016/j.ygcen.2017.07.010

Wittchen, H. U., Jacobi, F., Rehm, J., Gustavsson, A., Svensson, M., Jönsson, B., … Steinhausen, H. C. (2011). The size and burden of mental disorders and other disorders of the brain in Europe 2010. *European Neuropsychopharmacology: The Journal of the European College of Neuropsychopharmacology*, *21*(9), 655–679. doi:10.1016/j.euroneuro.2011.07.018

World Health Organization. (2005). *Mental health: Facing the challenges, building solutions*. Copenhagen: Author.

World Health Organization. (2012). *Understanding and addressing violence against women*. Geneva: Author. Retrieved from https://apps.who.int/iris/bitstream/handle/10665/77432/WHO_RHR_12.36_eng.pdf;jsessionid=5C773059CB125DDDC59803C90725148C?sequence=1

World Health Organization. (2020). *Mental health and psychosocial considerations during the COVID-19 outbreak*. Geneva: Author. Retrieved from https://www.who.int/docs/default-source/coronaviruse/mental-health-considerations.pdf

Wright, K. (2017). Voices now reveals results of big choral census. *Rhinegold*. Retrieved from https://www.rhinegold.co.uk/choir_organ/voices-now-reveals-results-big-choral-census/

Wyss, J. D. (1812). *The Swiss Family Robinson (Der Schweizerische Robinson). Zürich: Orell, Füßli und Compagnie.*

Xiang, Y.-T., Yang, Y., Li, W., Zhang, Q., Cheung, T., & Ng, C. H. (2020). Timely mental health care for the 2019 novel coronavirus outbreak is urgently needed. *The Lancet Psychiatry*, 7(3), 228–229. doi:10.1016/S2215-0366(20)30046-8

Yi-Ling, L. (2020, June 5). Is Covid-19 changing our relationships? *BBC Future*. Retrieved from https://www.bbc.com/future/article/20200601-how-is-covid-19-is-affecting-relationships

YouGov. (2020). Britain's mood, measured weekly [Data set]. Retrieved from https://yougov.co.uk/topics/science/trackers/britains-mood-measured-weekly

Young, C. (2020, May 5). More than food banks are needed to feed the hungry during the coronavirus pandemic. *The Conversation*. Retrieved from https://theconversation.com/more-than-food-banks-are-needed-to-feed-the-hungry-during-the-coronavirus-pandemic-136164

Zavaleta, D., Samuel, K., & Mills, C. (2014). *Social isolation: A conceptual and measurement proposal.* OPHI Working Papers 67. Retrieved from https://www.ophi.org.uk/wp-content/uploads/ophi-wp-67.pdf

Zhang, S. X., Wang, Y., Jahanshahi, A. A., Li, J., & Schmitt, V. G. H. (2020). Mental distress of adults in Brazil during the COVID-19 crisis. *medRxiv*. doi:10.1101/2020.04.18.20070896

Zweig, S. (1941). *Chess. (A. Bell, Trans.). Translated in English. Originally published as Schachnovelle.* London: Penguin Classics, 2017.

INDEX